THE

ROTATION

DIET

ALSO BY MARTIN KATAHN, PHD

The T-Factor Diet

The T-Factor Fat Gram Counter (with Jaime Pope)

THE
ROTATION
DIET

Martin Katahn, PhD

W. W. Norton & Company
New York * London

For information about permission to reproduce selections from this book,
write to Permissions, W. W. Norton & Company, Inc.,
500 Fifth Avenue, New York, NY 10110

For information about special discounts for bulk purchases, please contact
W. W. Norton Special Sales at specialsales@wwnorton.com or 800-233-4830

Manufacturing by LSC Harrisonburg
Book design by Chris Welch
Production manager: Louise Mattarelliano

Library of Congress Cataloging-in-Publication Data
Katahn, Martin.
The rotation diet / Martin Katahn.
p. cm.
Includes bibliographical references and index.
ISBN 978-0-393-34131-7 (pbk.)
1. Low-calorie diet. 2. Low-calorie diet—Recipes. I. Title.
RM222.2.K347 2012
641.5'63—dc23
2011044035

W. W. Norton & Company, Inc.
500 Fifth Avenue, New York, N.Y. 10110
www.wwnorton.com

W. W. Norton & Company Ltd.
15 Carlisle Street, London W1D 3BS

2 3 4 5 6 7 8 9 0

Contents

1 WHAT'S IT ALL ABOUT?   9

2 THE 200-CALORIE SOLUTION: Gaining Control over Your Metabolism   19

3 HOW THE ROTATION DIET CAME INTO BEING: A Personal Success Story   29

4 HOW THE ROTATION DIET CAME INTO BEING: History and Research   39

5 KNOW THE ENEMY, WIN THE WAR   49

6 GETTING STARTED ON THE RIGHT FOOT   61

7 THE ROTATION DIET FOR WOMEN AND MEN   72

   Recipes   101

8 APPLYING THE 200-CALORIE SOLUTION TO DAILY LIFE   161

9   TAKING A VACATION FROM DIETING:
    The Transition to Maintenance   188

10 WEIGHT MAINTENANCE: A Lifetime Challenge   203

11 ALTERNATE MENUS FOR THE ROTATION DIET   232

    Recipes   259

12 EPILOGUE   297

Acknowledgments   299

Appendix A: Calorie, Fat Gram, and Fiber Counter   303

Appendix B: Body Mass Index   357

Resources   361

The Rotation Diet Pocket Edition for Women   367

The Rotation Diet Pocket Edition for Men   377

Index   387

THE
ROTATION
DIET

1

WHAT'S IT ALL ABOUT?

n February 1986, seventy-five thousand people in Nashville, Tennessee, joined together, all with the same thing in mind: to lose weight using the Rotation Diet. Over a period of three weeks, crowds of eager Nashvillians picked up instructions for the diet at Kroger supermarkets and weighed in there on a weekly basis. During the rest of the year, fifteen million more people picked up Rotation Diet pamphlets at thousands of supermarkets around the United States. When the first edition of *The Rotation Diet*, complete with menus and recipes, was published, three million copies were sold.

The average weight loss during the supermarket promotion replicated almost exactly what the research team had obtained in the study at the Vanderbilt Weight Management Program (WMP): Women lost an average of *two-thirds of a pound per day for twenty-one days*. Some women, especially heavier women who were retaining water, lost as much as a pound a day, two to three inches around the waist in just three days, and one to three dress or pant sizes in three weeks. All in all, approximately 1,000,000 pounds were shed in Nashville, and untold millions more were lost around the United States.

So, if people can lose weight so quickly and easily on the Rotation Diet, why bother to update and revise it? If you have dieted in the past and regained weight afterward, like the vast majority of people who go on *any* reducing diet do, you already know the answer: dieting does only half the job! *It's one thing to lose the weight. It's quite another to keep it off.*

Losing weight and maintaining that loss for the rest of your life pose a number of different issues. In this new, revised edition of *The Rotation Diet*, I propose to show you how to do the complete job. I know how to do this. Forty-eight years ago I lost 75 pounds, and I have not regained a single pound. I know how to keep the weight off and can tell you how to do it too.

So, if you are like 90 to 95 percent of all overweight people who go on a reducing diet and lose weight only to gain it back again, I can tell you how to prevent rebounding. Most of us have some behaviors or environmental influences that must be changed in order to stay healthy and slim.

Research has shown that successful people find their own, unique way of weight management. For myself, and for about 95 percent of people who succeed in long-term weight management, one of the keys to success is to increase one's daily energy expenditure to the tune of at least 200 calories. Why are those 200 calories so important to weight management? *Because that's the energy expenditure it takes to keep 25 pounds of fat, once lost, from sneaking back into your fat cells!* Do you have more than 25 pounds to lose? Let me reassure you, I can show you from personal experience that losing the second 25 pounds can be as easy as losing the first.

Perhaps the easiest way to burn these extra calories is to walk for 30 to 40 minutes a day. Up until now I did not think there were any other ways that came close to the effectiveness of walking as the key to weight maintenance. But there are, and I discuss them later in the book. One of them, or combinations of them, should fit you and your lifestyle.

If you follow my suggestions over the next few weeks, a few months from now you will wonder why you didn't discover how to keep those pounds off before. Truly, it's easier than you think.

THE ROTATION METHOD OF
WEIGHT MANAGEMENT

More and more professionals in the weight-management field have come to realize that when people need to lose more than 10 to 15 pounds, moderate caloric restriction in their diet for many weeks on end often becomes both discouraging and depressing. After several weeks of slow, gradual weight loss, they hit plateaus, and a single deviation from the diet (a single high-calorie meal, a salty dish or snack) leads to a demoralizing increase in weight, mainly due to water retention. Instead, many professionals who recommend slow, gradual weight loss now suggest a time-limited plan, for example, no longer than three months at a time. In this way people find it easier to maintain their motivation (and their spirits) during the designated period.

The first persons to try out the Rotation Diet in the WMP were four women in a group of eighteen who were halfway through one of our standard ten-week programs in which we prescribed a 1200-calorie diet. They were discouraged because they hadn't lost as much weight as they had hoped. So I told them how I had lost weight myself on a rotation plan, and they volunteered to try it for three weeks. At the end of that time, their results caused a great deal of excitement. Weight loss increased significantly, as did morale!

We then organized a formal test group of twenty women who right from the start began their weight-loss program on the Rotation Diet. We found that the women on the Rotation Diet lost, on average, as much weight in three weeks (12½ pounds) as persons who had participated in our standard ten-week programs. Eighteen (90 percent) of the twenty women declared a preference for the Rotation Diet over a standard 1200-calorie diet.

USING THE ROTATION DIET

There are two basic ways to use the Rotation Diet to lose weight. One is to follow my lead. I never counted calories. I never kept an eating diary. I found an approach to dieting that actually made it fun, and I lost 75 pounds in a little over a year. I'll show you how you can adopt a similar approach if it appeals to you, as well as how I have kept all that weight off for so many years.

In contrast, we gave our research participants daily menus and recipes that were based on eating a specified amount of calories each day, plus free foods. It offers a caloric guarantee of an average loss of about 13 pounds in three weeks.

The women ate approximately 600 calories per day for three days, followed by 900 calories per day for four days, and then a week of 1200 calories per day, returning to the 600/900-calorie rotation once again. They had a diet consisting of a wide variety of foods.

Men had a core diet of more calories, approximately 1200 per day for the first three days, 1500 per day for the next four, followed by a week on 1800 calories per day. They repeated the 1200/1500 rotation for the final week.

However, you are not allowed to go hungry! I will provide you with a list of *free vegetables* and *safe fruits* to add to the core plan. These foods are so low in calories that even if you add as many as three to four servings a day, they will hardly slow your weight loss. The use of fruits for snacks and desserts should become a permanent part of your weight-maintenance plan too. In addition to helping you maintain your weight loss, they will greatly increase your diet's nutritional value.

When you finish the three-week rotation, *you MUST stop dieting.* You have to take a vacation! You will gradually add foods back into your diet in an experiment to see which of them helps with weight maintenance and which ones lead to extra pounds. If you have more weight to lose, before you repeat a rotation, this brief vacation of a week or a month or more (it's up to you) will not only increase your motivation to succeed, but also *help guarantee that you will not regain any weight when you reach your goal weight.* I'll explain the reasons in the next chapter, on gaining control over your metabolism.

In addition to more specific instructions on how to implement the dietary aspects of the Rotation Diet, I want to give you the advice we gave participants in the WMP when they met with us for weekly supervision and guidance. Successful weight management requires that you anticipate events, pressures, and temptations that might interfere with your resolve. There are folks in your life who, with or without malice, will get in the way of your success. The easy availability of high-calorie, appetite-stimulating foods, the multibillion-dollar industry peddling them, and the work-saving devices of modern technology that use electricity and gasoline to do the work your muscles once had to do, make the world around you very unfriendly to weight management. And unless you learn how to deal with "the devil within," there is a chance that well-ingrained lifestyle habits will lead you to become your own worst enemy.

In this book, I provide guidance on how to conquer your own impulses and how to deal with pressure to eat from others. For instance, you may be very fond of "junk" foods that contain almost no nutritional value other than calories, like candy, sweets, and salty chips. Or you may be just as fond of what I call "supernormal" foods. These foods have some nutritional value but are specially designed with blends of salt, fat, sugar, and creative flavorings to tempt you to overeat; they include cakes, cookies, and pies and the rich sauces used to dress up a main dinner entrée. Will it be possible to include them from time to time, after your three weeks on the diet, without gaining all your weight back? Yes, it will, and you will find that information later in this book.

Perhaps you have enough willpower to keep away from such foods on your own, but you don't know how to handle eating out or resisting a host's entreaties to try highly fattening foods at a party. This book gives you the advice that will allow you to go out, but not at the risk of adding on pounds.

Another important issue can be the way you have been talking to yourself about your efforts to control your appetite or to develop a more active lifestyle. You may have been overly hard on yourself, kicking yourself because of your past inability to control your weight. Such a self-derisive attitude is not helpful. While mistakes point out what you may be doing wrong, they don't show you what to do to be successful. The Rotation Diet breeds success, and success will give you something positive to talk to yourself about.

Throughout this book I describe the many strategies that other successful people have reported as being important to keeping weight off. Successful people find a way that fits their individual situations and personal tastes in food. They face the same difficulties you have faced before and will face in the future. I pay special attention to the published reports and individual stories from the National Weight Control Registry, in which over five thousand people describe how they lost at least 30 pounds and kept them off for at least a year.

In the first edition of *The Rotation Diet*, the Program's nutrition consultant developed alternate menus to illustrate how well you can eat on healthful weight-reducing and weight-maintenance diets. Over the years, my wife, daughter, and I have created scores of tasty new recipes, including vegetarian and low-salt ones. A number of these have been added to the original menus.

SPECIAL HEALTH BENEFITS OF THE ROTATION DIET

The Rotation Diet will not only lead to rapid weight loss. It has many other significant health benefits as well.

On average, there is a 10 percent reduction in serum cholesterol levels and a 15 percent reduction in circulating triglyceride levels, even in persons whose cholesterol and triglyceride levels are not abnormally high to begin with. Of course, the more elevated these levels were, the more benefit you can expect. (A high cholesterol level is a significant factor in cardiovascular disease, and high triglyceride levels have also been implicated.) Fasting glucose levels, if they were high, tend to return to normal so that if your doctor has said that you have "high blood sugar," there is every likelihood that it will normalize, and stay normal, if you follow my maintenance suggestions.

You will be interested in knowing that a large percentage of overweight persons with mild essential hypertension eliminate, or at least lower, their need for medication with the loss of only about 10 percent of their body weight. Thus, you don't even have to lose all your excess weight before you can obtain a significant health benefit from the Rotation Diet. Because salt (owing to its sodium content) can play a significant role in hypertension independent of its role in obesity, I have included a special section on how to reduce salt in your diet based my own recent experience. Additional benefits of losing weight can include a reduction in the severity of symptoms of depression, arthritis, and sleep apnea.

A final word of advice before you begin. One of the first rules of good practice in the health field requires that my advice not hurt anyone. We had a perfect record in the WMP and I want it to stay that way. While the Rotation Diet can be used in reasonable comfort by persons in good health, no one should undertake this or any other fast-weight-loss program without consulting with his or her physician. The menus for the 1200-calorie weeks are suitable for most diabetics, but recent research and practice have shown that there is no single correct diet to treat all diabetics. So if you are diabetic, it is especially important for you to discuss your situation with your physician. As I mentioned, if you have hypertension, your need for medication, including a diuretic, may be reduced or entirely eliminated in just a few weeks. That's a fantastic health benefit of the Rotation Diet. However, your medication must be monitored by your doctor during a diet. Do not make any changes in your medication without your doctor's supervision.

There are certain other important limitations in the use of the Rotation Diet in addition to the ones mentioned. The diet is not appropriate for children and adolescents, although if you show the menus for Week 2 for both men and women to your doctor or nutritionist, he or she will be able to suggest additions that will be suitable for your children. The diet is not suitable for women who are pregnant or nursing, or for people who are intensely active already—for example, persons who run several miles a day. In my opinion, active men and women should not cut more than 500 calories a day below their maintenance levels in order to lose weight and still maintain their health and energy levels.

Remember that this diet is meant to make you feel good. If the addition of the *free vegetables* and *safe fruit* that I suggest in Chapter 7 during the 600-calorie rotation are not enough food to keep you energetic and in good spirits, do not hesitate to increase your calories to 900, or even to 1200, if you are a woman. Men on the 1200-calories rotation should go up to 1500 or 1800 calories. Maintaining good health, mental and physical, during a diet is much more important than setting a weight-loss record.

The diet has been carefully designed with the Recommended Dietary Allowances of known vitamins and minerals in mind. One of our primary goals was to select foods that would maintain electrolyte balance (the correct ratio of potassium to sodium) over the entire period in which you would be on the Rotation Diet. If your physician or other health care providers have any questions about this diet, please have them make photocopies of the Rotation Diet Pocket Edition for Women (pages 367–76) or for Men (pages 377–86), for their close examination during your next visit. (They might like to hand copies out to their patients. Instructions for couples are also included in the Pocket Edition for Women.)

And now on to Chapter 2. Please do not begin the Rotation Diet before you have read Chapter 2.

2

THE 200-CALORIE
SOLUTION

Gaining Control over Your Metabolism

You are just 200 calories a day away from being permanently slimmer, healthier, and more totally alive. But it's not counting these calories that does it for you—you must burn them! As I said in Chapter 1, going on a diet solves only half of the weight-management problem. It's the easy half, and the Rotation Diet can do it for you safely and quickly. But I have to be blunt about it. You are not likely to keep the weight off if you try to control only your food intake. You must take charge of your life in such a way that you expend at least 200 calories more in physical activity—any activity that gets you moving—every day.

Why 200 calories? Because if you are 25 pounds overweight, 200 calories in your daily diet is being used just to keep your fat cells alive. Do you want to lose weight and be sure to keep it off? Do you want to be able to enjoy food and eat like "a normal human being"? Then, every day you must burn up the calories that keep those fat cells alive, and that led to your gaining weight in the first place. It's a lifetime job, but one you can do. Chapter 8 shows you how to expend that energy, starting off with a few minutes a day and working up to thirty to forty minutes, and it'll make it easy to become a habit.

Most overweight people do not fully appreciate how inactive they are. Many do not engage in outdoor activities and have never cultivated the basic skills to engage in sports, even as children. Video research has confirmed the relative lack of movement of obese adolescents during play. In a volleyball game with a group of overweight participants, I saw how some overweight folks would take a step toward the ball while it was in play, but if they missed or made an error, it was our average-weight staff assistants who raced about, chasing and bending to retrieve the ball and put it back in play. The staff enjoyed the exercise and didn't even think of slowing the pace and intensity of the game to match that of the slower participants. In a study of campers in the national parks, I found that obese people use equipment that requires less work, such as mobile homes rather than tents or tent trailers. Since 1960 the estimated mean daily energy expenditure attributable to work-related physical activity has dropped by more than 100 calories in both men and women in the United States. About half the population in the United States does not expend energy much above the resting metabolic level for a major part of their lives.

Research has shown many overweight people are on their feet or walking around for fewer than two miles a day. Many overweight people spend twenty-two hours or more every day either sitting or sleeping, not even standing. To figure out how much you actually walk, buy a pedometer or step counter, or simply count the time you spend standing or moving. This will give you a starting point to work from. (Pedometers and step counters are discussed in Chapter 8.)

Thin people move considerably more on average than over-weight people. In the same occupations, thin persons move two to three miles a day more than their heavier counterparts. Look around at your job site and see if that isn't true. Still, on average, even the amount that thin people move on the job compares poorly with that of our forebears. One hundred twenty-five years ago, just to get the job of living done, the average American was walking seven to eight miles a day, in addition to doing work that required more muscular involvement. People did not have to go out of their way to get some exercise. The automobile may be more responsible for the epidemic of obesity in this country than any other single technological advance, followed by the availability of electricity to power the tools that do the work we once had to do manually.

Most people overestimate the amount of walking done in various occupations and the amount they themselves do each day. When the WMP measured the amount of walking restaurant servers did during an eight-hour shift at a nearby popular sit-down restaurant, it added up to just two miles! They were on their feet, busily moving during breakfast and lunch times, but in between they were sitting (and eating). Much to my own surprise, I found that the total amount of walking I did while shopping in my local supermarket added up to just slightly over one-quarter of a mile. I increased the distance by parking at the farthest point in the store's parking lot.

HOW MUCH ENERGY DOES A PERSON NEED IN A DAY?

In January 2011, the U.S. Department of Agriculture (USDA) and Department of Health and Human Services (HHS) published the latest Estimates of Energy Requirements (EER) for men and women at a healthy weight at various ages. The amount of physical activity is calculated for sedentary, moderately active, and active lifestyles. The estimates are based on a "reference" woman, who is five feet four inches tall and weighs 126 pounds, and a "reference" man, who is five feet ten inches tall and weighs 154 pounds.*

At age nineteen, a sedentary woman at the reference height and weight needs, on average, 2000 calories per day, while a man at the reference height and weight needs 2600 calories. At age forty-six, estimated energy needs go down. The reference woman with a sedentary lifestyle will, on average, need 1800 calories a day, while the reference man will need 2200 calories. The lowering of energy needs, and thus calories, as we get older is mainly due to the loss of muscle mass that occurs with age. Also, even if we are moderately active or active, we tend toward the lower range of those categories as we age. (See Table 2-1.)

---

* Estimates for three different levels of physical activity—sedentary, moderately active, and active—are given. *Sedentary* means a lifestyle that includes only the light physical activity associated with typical day-to-day life. *Moderately active* means a lifestyle that includes physical activity equivalent to walking 1½ to 3 miles per day at 3 to 4 miles per hour, in addition to the light physical activity associated with typical day-to-day life. *Active* means a lifestyle that includes physical activity equivalent to walking more than 3 miles per day at 3 to 4 miles per hour, in addition to the light physical activity associated with typical day-to-day life. The entire Dietary Guidelines for Americans 2010 is available for download at www.dietaryguidelines.gov.

Table 2-1

Estimated Energy Needs (Calories) for Women Per Day			
	Sedentary	Moderately Active	Active
AGE 19–20	2000	2200	2400
AGE 46–50	1800	2000	2200
Estimated Energy Needs (Calories) for Men Per Day			
AGE 19–20	2600	2800	3000
AGE 46–50	2200	2400	2800

Participants in the WMP would voice disbelief and skepticism after seeing calorie levels such as those in Table 2-1. Some found it an alarmingly high number of calories: "If I ate 2000 calories a day I would be twice as fat as I am now." And "Those numbers don't apply to me. I can't lose weight on a diet of only 1200 calories a day. I've tried. I must have a slow metabolism."

In order to put the information in Table 2-1 in perspective, it helps to understand how your metabolism works.

THE REALITIES OF METABOLISM

If your weight has been steady for a period of time (say, several weeks), varying by only a few pounds up or down, you are considered to be in *energy balance*. That means the amount of energy (calories)* in the food you have eaten is equal to the amount of energy you have been burning during this time. During periods

---

* In measuring the energy in the food we eat, a calorie is the amount of heat required at sea level to raise the temperature of 1 kilogram (2.2 pounds) of water one degree Celsius (0.8 degree Fahrenheit).

of weight gain, you ate a greater amount of energy (calories) than you expended in daily activity. That extra energy became fat. At times when you lost weight, you took in less energy through your food than you needed each day. That deficiency was made up by withdrawing energy that had been stored in your fat cells.

Let's go a little further, explaining how your body uses calories, to give you a better understanding of your metabolism.

Resting Energy Expenditure

The *resting energy expenditure* (REE, sometimes referred to as the *resting metabolic rate*, or RMR) is the rate at which you burn calories when in your most restful state, such as when you are sleeping or quietly lying down. It's the number of calories your body burns up to keep your heart pumping, blood circulating, and your brain, liver, kidneys, and other body organs functioning. It can be expressed as the number of calories needed per pound of body weight or as the total caloric needs for these basic bodily functions for an entire day. For the reference woman, it would be around 10 calories per pound of body weight. If you totaled the amount of energy she needed for the entire day, you would take her weight (126 pounds) and multiply it by 10, the amount of calories for each pound of her weight. Thus, her basic needs (her REE) would be 1260 calories.

Activity and Energy Needs

The *activity part* of your energy needs each day is the cost of moving your body about to get the job of living done. In tables that estimate the amount of calories burned in various activities, these additional calories are added to the cost of just sitting still, reading, or watching TV.* For example, the energy expended in walking three miles per hour is about three times the energy used in sitting still. If you are constantly moving your arms while sitting and doing your job (think of a cellist), you will be expending about twice the energy of sitting still. Working at the computer, however, requires hardly more energy than sitting still. Typing on a manual typewriter required 15 percent more energy than typing on a keyboard does today.

Thermic Effect of Food

In addition to the energy cost of your vital bodily functions and the activity part of your energy expenditure, there is the energy cost of converting the calories and other nutrients in the food you eat into the form your body can use. This is referred to as the *thermic effect of food* (TEF), which is the heat produced by the body in metabolizing your food. It generally adds up to a bit less than 10 percent of the calories in the food itself. For example, the reference woman, who is consuming 2000 calories per day, would use a little less than 200 calories per day in metabolizing her food.

There is very little you can do about the thermic effect of food associated with your diet. You can give it a small kick by drinking a glass of ice water (the body spends a few calories warming it to body temperature and moving the ½ pound it adds temporarily to your body weight) or eating hot peppers (which raise body

---

* See Table 8-1, on energy expenditures in various activities, page 169. Sitting still reading or watching TV burns up about 10 percent more calories than quietly lying down or sleeping.

temperature a bit; you know it's happening if your scalp begins to tingle and sweat). However, the impact of such foods in your diet is quite insignificant compared to the impact changes in your lifestyle can make on your total daily energy needs. (In Chapter 9 I explain how you can make a more significant impact on your weight by increasing the fiber in your diet.)

Another factor in determining your REE and your total daily energy expenditure is the difference between fat and muscle tissue. Fat tissue is relatively inactive and takes considerably less energy than muscle tissue to stay alive. Let's go back to our reference woman to see what this means practically.

As we saw before, the reference woman, weighing 126 pounds, has a daily REE of 1260 calories. Another woman, of the same age and height, but who weighs 50 pounds more—176 pounds—will need only 8½ calories per pound to cover her resting energy needs because her added weight is composed of relatively inactive fat cells. Her REE is her total body weight (176 pounds) multiplied by the energy she uses per pound of body weight (8½ calories), which equals 1496 calories. That's 236 calories more than her thinner counterpart to maintain her weight of 176 pounds.

You see how this can become confusing. Looked at per pound of body weight, it seems as if the heavier woman has a "slow metabolism," requiring only 8½ calories per pound of body weight compared with 10 calories per pound in the reference woman. However, with regard to her total daily REE, she actually needs 19 percent more calories to keep her vital functions working compared to the woman who weighs 126 pounds.

The energy expended in physical activity also varies with body weight. Just as it takes more gas to move a loaded 1½-ton pickup truck than one without its load, it takes more energy for a person to move a heavier body than a lighter one. Walking at three miles per hour, a person weighing 176 pounds may expend about a calorie a minute more than a person weighing 126 pounds. For the heavier person, this amounts to burning about 60 calories more per hour of walking at three miles per hour.

THE EFFECT OF WEIGHT LOSS ON YOUR METABOLISM AND DAILY ENERGY NEEDS

Comparing the extra energy required to move a heavy body with the energy required to move a light body also works in reverse! As you lose weight, your body requires less and less energy to move about. Your smaller body will also decrease its resting energy needs (although you can compensate to some extent by adding muscle tissue, which will happen if you follow the suggestions in Chapter 8). Fortunately, having a smaller body makes it easier to move around, and you may even find yourself being more active spontaneously.

For each pound of weight you lose, your metabolic rate goes down by about 8 calories. If you lose 25 pounds, it means that your total daily energy needs will decrease by around 200 calories. Sound familiar? If you don't want your pounds back, but still want to keep your food intake close to where it is today, you have to find a way to expend 200 calories every day.

THE STARVATION RESPONSE: ANOTHER THING TO WORRY ABOUT?

No! At the time I wrote the first edition of *The Rotation Diet*, extremely low-calorie liquid diets were the rage. Some of these diets contained only 400 calories a day and were sometimes used for weeks on end. If you were to go on such a diet, after several weeks, acting as if you might be starving, your body would go into "conservation mode." Your metabolism would slow dramatically, maybe down by 40 or even 50 percent below its non-dieting rate. The resting energy needs of our 176-pound woman on this diet might decrease from a total of 1496 calories per day to only half that, or just 748 calories per day.

You can imagine what happens when people on liquid diets of this sort begin eating normal food again. They begin to *gain* weight rapidly on just 1000 to 1100 calories a day. It may take weeks or months before resting energy needs return to near-normal levels.

I was particularly anxious to determine if the Rotation Diet would have such an impact on our WMP participants. Before starting them on the diet, we measured their REE. Then, we measured it weekly during the three-week rotation. Based on my own three-week experience in losing weight and keeping it off, I had expected—and hoped—that such very brief periods of low-calorie dieting, combined with the increase in physical activity, would prevent any decrease in the REE. Happily, I was right. We found not even the slightest deleterious effect. In fact, we actually found a slight (but statistically insignificant) increase in metabolic rate. I can say with confidence that when you use the Rotation Diet, the impact on your metabolism will be no greater than that of a person who loses weight at a slow 1 to 1½ pounds per week.

In Chapter 3, you will find out how I lost weight on the diet that led to the Rotation Diet, how I increased my physical activity and never gained the weight back.

3

HOW THE ROTATION DIET
CAME INTO BEING

A Personal Success Story

Forty-eight years ago I weighed 75 pounds more than I do today. The way I lost that weight and kept it off forms my personal basis for *The Rotation Diet*. I'm proud of what I have accomplished in managing my own weight, and I think you can do it just as well. So I'd like to tell you something about myself and how I did it.

I was one of those fat kids who had no memory of ever being thin. Instead, I have memories such as not being able to run fast enough to keep up with my playmates, being chosen last for all of the games that required physical movement, and being so fat by age four or five that I couldn't even bend over in my snowsuit to make snowballs. I found some small consolation in comparing myself with another "little" fat boy. I used to repeat to myself, "I'm not the fattest boy in the class. John is fatter than I am." Perhaps poor John was consoling himself in a similar way, using me for comparison.

By the time I was twelve years old, I was 50 pounds overweight. My parents became so concerned that they took me to the pediatrician for a visit I will never forget. Dr. Davis measured my body frame, and to this day, in my mind's eye, I can see him clearly, standing before me, running his finger along the diagonal of a chart, reaching the corner, looking down at me, emitting a surprised little chuckle, and saying, "You aren't even on the chart!"

I have fond memories of my childhood doctor even though I did not lose weight as a result of any of his efforts. I always had the feeling that he was trying to help me. After the appropriate tests, he determined that my thyroid hormone levels were low and I had a slow metabolic rate. He placed me on thyroid medication and gradually increased the dosage up to four grains as I gradually, in turn, upped my consumption of potato salad. He told my parents that they should encourage me to restrict my food intake, which they always did, but only after reminding me of the starving kids in Armenia (my parents were lucky enough to have left Russia in the late nineteenth century). I paid more heed to the needs of the starving kids in Armenia while I was eating than to my parents' admonitions to restrain myself, which always seemed to follow after I had finished. In the end, I began to have heart palpitations, the thyroid medication had to be discontinued, and my parents gave up on their efforts to control my eating.

By the time I reached thirty-five, I was 75 pounds overweight and suffered from hypertension. I remember the day when I had to lie down on a couch for an hour to bring my blood pressure down to normal so that the examining physician would okay me for an insurance policy to cover the new home I had just purchased upon moving to Nashville. And I certainly know the effort that is involved in lugging all that extra fat around! I would get out of breath just going across the street from my office and walking up one flight of stairs to the library. I remember putting off library visits until I had several tasks to do, because of the effort involved in getting there and walking up and down between the stacks. My weight, inactivity, and genetic predisposition also blessed me with varicose veins by the time I was twelve. At that early age, I had my first attack of thrombophlebitis, which led to the injection treatment that was popular seventy years ago and which resulted in permanent injury and disfigurement to one of my legs. Every two or three years I would suffer another attack, at times requiring me to spend as long as a month either in bed or sitting with my leg elevated, and another month or so on crutches. Unfortunately, no physician was able to prescribe the treatment that finally ended this plague of inflammations and clotting. While becoming a tennis player was my key to weight management, it was only after I added jogging two to five miles a day beginning at the age of fifty that the problem was remedied.

Of course I tried many diets during my early years. I tried grapefruit diets and egg diets. I tried fasting and even devised my own version of a high-protein, powdered diet. I would stuff gigantic capsules with gelatin and swallow a package worth of capsules with two glasses of water for breakfast, and another package worth of capsules for lunch, with yet another two glasses of water. (You can imagine what I did for the rest of the day.) I could lose weight as fast as anyone. And put it back on just as fast.

The turning point finally happened while I was playing a game of Ping-Pong outside my office in the hallway of the Psychology Department, where we had set up a makeshift table. I began to get dizzy and nauseated, I broke out in a cold sweat, I could not catch my breath, and my knees began to quiver. Somehow I made it back to a chair in my office, but I did not want to face reality: I was having a heart attack. I did not want to face it even though I had been having chest pains periodically for several years. I did not want to face it even though one time I had actually been knocked off my feet by the pain and unable to lift my arm.

I gradually returned to near normal in about forty-five minutes. I called my wife first, to tell her what had happened and to assure her that I felt all right but that I was going to a doctor. The cardiogram did indeed suggest that I had had a heart attack, and I am forever grateful to Dr. Ed Tarpley for the treatment he prescribed. With cardiogram in hand, Ed said simply, "Dick, you've got to lose that weight. I don't care what diet you use, but you have got to get active. That is the only way you will keep the weight off and possibly prevent another occurrence."

The clearest thing in my memory of the days that followed is the recurring thought that I wanted to stay alive as my children grew up. My daughter was eight and my son ten. And it was no time to leave my wife—our love and friendship have always been very special, and then, as always, we had so much to look forward to together. Would I finally find a way to take the weight off in spite of all of my past failures? Would I be able to keep it off? I had no successful past behavior to guide me since there never was a time in my life when I had been thin. And could I find an activity that wouldn't hurt my legs and put me in bed with thrombophlebitis every other year? At that time, too much walking or the slightest bruise could do it. I knew no active games. I didn't even know what the inside of a gym might look like, and I certainly was not going to get inside one and undress so that everyone could see how fat I was.

Back in 1963 I did not know as much about the design of a diet for weight loss as I do now. (I was researching the effects of anxiety on learning and the treatment of phobias. The WMP did not come into existence until 1976.) I did know one thing at that time, however, and that was—*something had to change!* You can't eat fatty foods and lots of sweets, consume alcohol, and lose weight easily. While I never overindulged in alcohol, after just a couple of drinks my pleasant celebratory mood could lead to overindulgence in general.

So, I cut them all out. *ALL*. For periods of three weeks I was absolutely perfect. Then I would *stop* dieting and return to my normal eating pattern, which included some things we all seem to prefer in our diets, like desserts and a glass of wine. I never regained any of the weight I had lost. Without my realizing it, the principles that would form the basis of the Rotation Diet twenty-two years after my heart attack were born.

What exactly was I doing and what had I learned? Here are a few of the main things:

First, I was following a quick-weight-loss plan that resulted in 15 to 20 pounds of weight loss each time I dieted.

Second, I never planned to diet more than three weeks at a time (with a week of careful transition back to a more normal eating pattern).

Third, I gradually increased my activity level (tennis became my activity of choice).

Fourth, by being active and not dieting for more than three weeks at a time, I evidently did not lower my metabolic rate, nor did I increase the fat storage ability that seems to follow prolonged use of a low-calorie diet, because I never regained any weight after each period of weight loss.

Fifth, before going on each weight-loss rotation, I would get really motivated to be *perfect*, knowing that 15 or more pounds were about to come off and that I intended to stop after three weeks. (I must admit that I once continued to diet for an extra week because I found it very hard to stop at three when I was being so successful in losing weight.)

SO WHAT DID I EAT ON MY ROTATION DIET?

What do I mean by *perfect* in describing the way I went about dieting? I quit eating all of the foods that I knew contributed to my obesity. I cut out all fried foods and desserts other than fruit. I cut out all alcohol, candy, cookies, cakes, pies, ice cream, all fatty and salty snacks (like potato and corn chips), and soft drinks. *In other words, I went "cold turkey"* except for the bit of butter I might add to toast or to cooked vegetables, and the half-and-half I added to my coffee. (I do not use butter and cream at all today.)

I never felt deprived, perhaps because my choice of *safe fruit* as a snack kept me from feeling hungry, and the weight-loss results were so dramatic!

Here are some examples of the meals I contrived to keep me happy. I alternated between several menus for breakfast, which I always ate at home.

1. 2 slices of dry toast (whole grain, rye, or pumpernickel) sometimes with jelly (little or no butter), coffee or tea, and a piece of fruit or a glass of juice, which I might save for later in the morning.
2. Cold cereal, with fruit and low-fat milk.
3. A slice of toast with one or two soft- or hard-boiled eggs, coffee, and juice with the meal or later in the morning.

For lunch I had to find a place that would make exactly what I wanted every day because it was more convenient to eat out than to prepare something to take to the office. The Campus Grill had just what I wanted. For five days a week, I ate one of two lunches.

1. My most frequent lunch was the dieter's special that was popular in those days: ground beefsteak (it was really just a large, lean hamburger patty, no more than 4 or 5 ounces, cooked weight), a scoop of cottage cheese (probably full-fat version), and usually sliced tomato and lettuce but sometimes a small dinner salad, coleslaw (it was ½ cup of the creamy version, but I don't recall it being overly fatty), or canned fruit. The meal came with a small roll on the side, which I ate plain, without butter.

2. For variety, once or twice a week I would have "soup of the day" (chicken noodle, vegetable or vegetable beef, tomato, etc.; these were all canned, individual servings heated to order) and a house salad. It came with two small packets of saltines. Sometimes I skipped the soup and had a large salad. At first I used the whole packet of dressing that came with it, but then I learned to just dip the tines of a fork in my salad dressing. It amazed me how little it took to make salad greens taste good. Even today I still order salad dressing on the side, and never end up eating more than half the serving.

Dinner at home almost always followed the same formula: a standard serving of either meat (for example, a London broil or a well trimmed rib-eye steak), poultry, or fish; a cooked vegetable; rice or potatoes; and sometimes a salad. This is when I discovered that I could enjoy a baked potato with just salt and pepper. Sometimes I would substitute a slice or two of whole-grain bread for the cooked starch. Dessert was either fresh or dried fruit, or, on occasion, one of my favorites at the time: two fig bars.

Today, as a fish-eating vegetarian, I would design two basic lunches a little differently for a diet like this. I would keep my soup-and-salad lunch similar to what it was in 1963, only I would stick with plant-based soups. Since I don't eat red meat or poultry, for my dieter's special I would substitute broiled or poached fish, a bowl of vegetarian chili, or a veggie-style burger, like Morning-Star Farms Grillers Original.

For dinner, I would replace the meat and poultry selections with fish and legume recipes, like the ones you will find in the recipe sections of this book.

Also, today there are many frozen-food entrées that fit this approach to reducing caloric intake. Check out Healthy Choice, Smart Ones, Lean Cuisine, and South Beach Living.

DEALING WITH SOCIAL SITUATIONS

At the start of my diet, I had some fears about how I would handle temptations that might occur when eating out in fine restaurants with friends. Our group of friends always enjoyed cocktails and wine with a festive dinner, and the test came quite early on in my diet.

One evening, while we were out to dinner with friends at a steak house, I had started off with a shrimp cocktail, followed by a steak and salad. My companions remarked on my "control"—I had passed on the hot bread and butter and had been sipping my glass of ice water as they enjoyed their cocktails. They asked me what diet I was using, and my answer just popped out, without much planning, because I had just noticed that everything I had been eating began with the letter *s*: "It's my own diet. I call it the 4S-Diet, and it's unlimited indulgence in shrimp, steak, salad, and sex."

The name of my diet got a few laughs, and since everyone began to notice that I was losing weight quickly, I began to respond to all subsequent questions about what diet I was on with, "The 4S-Diet." My description was always worth a chuckle or two, but I soon discovered that it was worth much, much more than a little laugh. It disarmed potential tempters and temptresses. *No one ever, at any party, dinner, or other social engagement, pushed me to deviate from my diet once I made my statement.* So I found it very easy to adhere to it, sticking, in reality, not just to my four *S*'s but to a wide variety of fruits, vegetables, lean meats, fish, and fowl.

I learned much, much more about successful weight loss as I began to implement my plan. The insights I gained made it relatively easy—much easier than I had expected. Many things that I did not actually plan or anticipate helped me lose 75 pounds in a little over a year. I will tell you all about these things in the book as I go along, showing step by step how I and other successful people actually implement the Rotation Diet. What I learned by chance and trial and error you can do intentionally.

As I write these words, I am in my eighty-third year. I was even able to quit smoking cigars in 1983 without re-gaining weight, and I have never had another heart attack. I have not spent a single day in bed with either an inflammation or a blood clot in my legs after I discovered what it takes to prevent their occurrence (losing weight and performing activities like walking and gentle jogging).

Losing weight and becoming active forty-eight years ago solved my blood pressure problem up until seven years ago, when my familial disposition to hypertension reappeared. I immediately solved the problem by cutting the amount of sodium in my diet. Since too much sodium in a diet can be an important health risk, right along with being overweight, I talk more about this in Chapter 7.

4

HOW THE ROTATION DIET CAME INTO BEING
History and Research

I n the early 1970s a young graduate student named Gordon Kaplan asked my advice on doing a study to investigate the behavioral approach to losing weight. Gordon had lost 100 pounds following advice that had begun to appear in the treatment literature. The adviser he was working with said he knew little about the area, and suggested he talk with me since I, too, had lost a lot of weight a number of years before.

His idea appealed to me, but since I had lost my weight in my own idiosyncratic cold-turkey way, I told him I needed to study the research that had so impressed him and the strategies that had been so effective in his own case. I also suggested we get our feet wet by working together using behavioral strategies to help some overweight people lose weight.

Several overweight graduate students from other departments in the university answered our announcement that we were available to offer counseling to anyone with a weight problem. For the next several months we acted as co-therapists, learning how to teach them the procedures used in the field and designing Gordon's study.

Gordon wanted as his research subjects people among the general public who were overweight and truly representative of persons who were joining weight-loss programs in our area. He arranged an interview with the women's editor of *The Tennessean*, Nashville's daily newspaper. In response to the interview, she wrote an article about the research that appeared on the front page of the women's section in the Sunday edition. By Wednesday we had signed up forty research subjects and had five hundred people on a waiting list! Gordon called the approach he was using "weight management" rather than referring to it as a program in weight control or weight loss. I believe he was among the first to use that term, if not the very first. It has become a common way to refer to programs that offer help to overweight persons.

Gordon gathered his data over a three-month period and then left for an internship, leaving me receiving several calls daily from folks on the waiting list. I called my other graduate students together and invited Dr. Ken Wallston, a professor in the medical school with a research interest in obesity, to join us. We agreed that the issue of obesity was a serious one, and that the area was ripe for continued research. We also felt the need to get financial support for the research, and the first study for which we submitted a grant to the National Institute of Mental Health was to investigate the helper therapy principle in weight management. We wanted to determine whether people who have received help in solving their own weight problems gain additional value by helping others. The answer is yes, and we put that idea to work in the WMP in the years that followed. When we submitted the research grant, we did not give the program a title other than to indicate that it was a study on weight management. It was the director of the grants management office at Vanderbilt University who suggested that we identify ourselves as the Vanderbilt Weight Management Program, and until my retirement in 1991, I was its director. After my retirement, the program was closed to the public, and those connected with it moved over to other units of the university. The program was continued, but it was limited to faculty and staff, who in turn developed programs for Vanderbilt students. At the present time weight-management classes are offered at the Kim Dayani Health Promotion Center at Vanderbilt University.

THE ORIGINAL WEIGHT MANAGEMENT PROGRAM

The original WMP employed sound nutritional principles. Leaders taught the participants how to keep eating and activity records. We recommended a balanced diet of 1200 calories a day for women and 1500 for men. We rehearsed behavior-modification strategies for modifying the eating environment and controlling eating behavior. We included several features in the program that helped participants maintain their weight loss, and since these can be helpful to everyone, I'll talk more about them in Chapter 10.

On the plus side, in comparison with the weight loss and *weight maintenance* obtained in most weight-control programs based on behavior modification, the WMP was doing quite well before we introduced the Rotation Diet. Over 32 percent of all participants in the WMP were in the desirable weight range for as long as three years after their participation. Twenty percent of the persons who had 40 pounds or more to lose did lose 40 pounds and were keeping it off. Based on our group averages, 85 percent of the weight that was lost during the program was being kept off. Yearly questionnaires showed that participants were eating a more nutritional diet than they had before participating in the WMP, and by and large, they were more active.

Compared with any other results over a three-year period of which we were aware, these were excellent. Losing just 5 to 10 percent of your weight has significant benefits to your health.

On the minus side, however, when we looked at the weight-loss records of thousands of persons (including participants in the WMP as well as reports in the literature for programs like ours), we saw that the average weight loss on such slow-weight-reducing diets for women was only about 1 to 1½ pounds per week. The average weight loss for programs all around the United States lasting ten weeks ranged between 10 and 15 pounds, just as it does today!

While a loss of 5 to 10 percent of body weight for a person who is 40 or 50 pounds or even more overweight can have significant health benefits, I sometimes get the feeling that health professionals use modest expected-loss figures such as these because they assume persons trying to lose weight will not do any better. They are preparing participants to be satisfied with less than they expect or would like.

The problem with gradual-weight-loss programs is that most persons find it difficult, if not impossible, to follow the slow, moderate approach for very long. There are too many choices to make, we are surrounded by tempting high-calorie foods, and our family and outside social lives continually expose us to temptations that are hard to resist for more than a short period of time. Most of us can be "pretty good" for short periods, but in a matter of weeks, say even three or four, we begin to make those tiny deviations, followed by larger deviations, that bring our weight losses to a virtual standstill.

All of this means that the true focus of our past success, and of programs that use moderate approaches, has been, and will continue to be, with a small percentage of persons who do not have very much weight to lose. Ten pounds—good. Twenty or twenty-five pounds—still pretty good. Of persons with more than that to lose, only a few can actually expect to make it to the "normal (healthy) weight" given in Appendix B if they use a slow, moderate approach to weight loss.

Considerations such as these kept me looking for ways to help people lose *more* weight and lose it *faster*, so that they would be inclined to remain motivated for whatever period it would take to be as successful as possible.

THE ROTATION DIET IS BORN

As I pondered different approaches to increasing the rate and total amount of weight our participants would lose, I kept returning to the method I had used myself (at that time, twenty-two years before): quick losses for three-week periods and then a "time-out." My daily activity kept me from regaining weight. Then, when the spirit moved me, another rotation. It's true that "my way" of losing weight did not follow the guidelines that are part of "standard practice" in nutrition, then and now, and my way was not what we had been encouraging our participants in the WMP to follow.

But I did lose 75 pounds and have kept them off for forty-eight years. How can you argue with such results? Had my way hurt me? On the contrary, I have been more successful than all but a handful of the persons who have followed standard practice. My way had no deleterious impact on my metabolism. My blood pressure today is in the healthy range, I am not diabetic, and I need no medication other than an aspirin or acetaminophen to relieve the aches associated with arthritis. And just in case you suffer from arthritis, I have some special advice for you on activity in Chapter 8.

Before I introduced my way to lose weight and keep it off to the WMP back in 1984, my major fear was that not everyone would have the beneficial results I had experienced. However, many respected professionals all over the country were coming to the same realization I had: traditional dietary means, even when combined with the best that behavioral psychology had to offer, were not leading to very much weight loss in the people who needed to lose more than 10 or 15 pounds. Many of these professional health workers were beginning to experiment with very-low-calorie diets, including powdered formula diets with as low as 400 to 600 calories a day for periods of up to two months, in an effort to find more effective weight-loss strategies. I did not want to use such diets because of the possibility of serious metabolic consequences. (They also can have serious effects on cardiac function and require constant medical supervision.) And I had personally seen the rapid gain in weight that almost invariably follows the use of such diets. Finally something occurred that convinced me to create what became known as the Rotation Diet.

We were halfway through one of our ten-week programs during the fall and winter of 1984–85 when four of the eighteen women in one of my groups expressed their great frustration with the rate of weight loss on our usual 1200-calorie diet. They were doing fine with their physical activity, but they were having trouble designing their own menus when they could include whatever they liked as long as they did not exceed 1200 calories a day.

So I laid out my plan to create a three-week quick-weight-loss diet with a period of rest, similar to what I had done many years before. The women were extremely eager to try it. We would monitor their metabolic rates on a weekly basis to determine whether or not a dramatic, but temporary, decrease in calories would lower their rates, which until that time had not declined.

You know the results. Although weight loss speeded up significantly, we could detect no decrease in metabolic rate. Morale skyrocketed, and their motivation to continue with their weight-loss program was restored. These results encouraged me to plan a much larger trial for the spring into the summer of 1985.

We recruited twenty women, who began right off with three days on a 600-calorie diet, four days at 900 calories, and then one week at 1200. They repeated the 600/900-calorie rotation in the third week. They were told to use *free vegetables* and to choose a *safe fruit* to supplement the core diet, so as never to be uncomfortably hungry. Most participants added three or four servings of vegetables and fruit each day to the core plan. Physical activity (walking or its equivalent in terms of energy expenditure) was gradually increased, with a goal of fifteen minutes per day the first week, moving up to forty-five minutes per day during the third week. We also set a target of activity for a minimum of five days each week, although we preferred six or seven provided it felt good! We obtained pre-program baseline resting metabolic rates, and then we monitored these rates on a weekly basis. We also obtained answers to a set of questions that measured the ease of sticking with the plan and satisfaction with progress. Of course, we were eager to compare the speed of weight loss with the 1- to 1½-pound weekly loss that is usually obtained with the 1200-calorie diets.

RESULTS WITH THE FIRST CLINICAL TRIAL USING THE ROTATION DIET

The women were able to stick closely to the plan, and the average weight loss was 12½ pounds in twenty-one days. That's about two-thirds of a pound a day. The heaviest women lost as much as a pound a day. There was no reduction in resting metabolic rate; in fact, there was a small (but statistically insignificant) metabolic increase. Ninety percent of the women said they preferred the Rotation Diet to the lower, more moderate diets they had tried in the past, and I even had a great deal of difficulty persuading some of them to take the at-least-one-week vacation from dieting that is an essential part of the plan.

SOME PERSONAL REACTIONS TO THE ROTATION DIET

To formally monitor reactions to the diet each week, we had participants fill out a questionnaire. Here are some of the written responses:

"It's so clear. You can't make a mistake!"

"It works!"

"The 600/900 is easy to stay on—fewer choices, fewer temptations."

"Very happy with this diet plan. Can't think of anything bad to say about it."

"The best thing about this diet is that I feel thinner (and better)."

"I am really having a good time on my walks. When I've lost weight before I've found it difficult to lose in my hips and thighs, but because of the walking this is the first place I'm losing. I've already gone down one entire dress size, and two in pant size. I love it."

"The best—plenty to eat and pleasant variety of foods [on 1200-calorie segment of the rotation]."

"When I reach the 1200 calories per day I really feel *rewarded* for having been so good on the 600/900."

"I feel better and have more energy."

"It works, and I'm really building self-esteem."

"I see the results I started out to accomplish."

"The 600/900 part is even easier than I thought it could possibly be."

Obviously, with such outstanding results, we made the Rotation Diet a part of our regular weight-loss program for persons who preferred a quick-loss plan and did not have any physical condition that made its use unwise.

HOW CAN A QUICK-WEIGHT-LOSS PLAN LEAD TO PERMANENT WEIGHT MANAGEMENT?

Whether you follow my personal cold-turkey method, or the calorie-based version of the Rotation Diet, you will be sticking with a diet built entirely around the kind of food that must remain the core of a lifelong nutritious diet. You may find that during the transition to a maintenance diet, when you begin to add more and different foods to your basic diet, you can, indeed, add some high-calorie foods (desserts, alcohol, snacks other than fruit, etc.) without gaining weight. Instructions for making this transition are in Chapter 9. Much will depend on your having incorporated extra activity burning 200 calories a day.

But I have another very important reason for having you cut out high-calorie foods that have such appetite stimulators as sugar, fat, and salt, and to limit these nutrients in processed foods as well as in your own cooking. These nutrients lead to overeating and obesity. I'll discuss this as I begin the next chapter.

5

KNOW THE ENEMY, WIN THE WAR

For most overweight people, especially the obese, making permanent changes that result in losing enough weight to meet healthy guidelines, and keeping it off, has proved to be very difficult. In fact, in spite of the many dangers on the Kansas plains and in the western mountains in the mid-nineteenth century, the percentage of pioneers crossing the United States in their covered wagons who made it safely to California is much higher than the percentage of overweight people in the American eating environment today who make it to a healthy weight.*

What is it about our appetite that leads us to overeat to the point of becoming overweight and obese? Is there something about the American diet that bears a direct responsibility for the rapid increase in weight in the past two decades? And if you are looking to make a permanent change in your own eating habits to combat being overweight, what does the Rotation Diet have to

* See Appendix B (page 357) for the body mass index and determination of healthy weight.

offer that will help you do it more easily and effectively than other approaches to weight management?

WHY DO HUMANS HAVE A PREFERENCE FOR HIGH-FAT, SWEET, AND SALTY FOODS?

Humans are attracted to foods blended with fat, sugar, and salt. They don't have to be hungry to experience an urge to eat them. The very sight or thought of such food can stimulate the production of saliva and start the stomach juices flowing. This taste preference has a long evolutionary history in which it became a part of our genetic heritage as the human race faced periodic famine and infectious disease.

Ever since we, the human race, turned from hunting and gathering to agriculture for our food supply, we have faced frequent famines. In fact, two-thirds of the earth's population still faces serious food shortages approximately every two years. The World Health Organization is predicting that we are about to enter one of those periods in the developing nations next year. Only in the Western world, and only for the past few hundred years, has there been anything approaching a stable food supply. Because of our past experience with famine, genetic lines that tended to store body fat and that developed a preference for foods that could add fat quickly were favored.

Infectious disease played a similar selective role. Together with famine, infectious disease often prevented half of newborn infants from reaching their first birthdays. Before the era of antibiotics and immunization, resistance to infectious disease depended in part on the amount of body fat an individual possessed, since the metabolic rate goes up about 7 percent for each degree (Fahrenheit) of fever. With just 4 degrees of fever, energy needs are about 28 percent higher than normal. Thus, individuals with genetic tendencies to obesity, or who liked fatty foods and so had a few extra pounds of fat storage, were better able to fight disease.

Because in the past individuals who did not possess the capacity to store fat easily or who did not care for fatty foods had less of a chance to reach reproductive age, we tend to be a species with rather strong tendencies to obesity given the availability of high-fat foods, especially when blended with the appropriate amounts of sugar and salt.

We learn which foods taste good through early experience in our food environments. Every culture in which fat, sugar, and salt are freely available at low cost has developed its own versions of foods that lead to overeating. Babies come to prefer salt in their food by the age of six months. We learn which foods can turn on our appetite through pairing the food—its sight, taste, and smell—with cues in the environment. It's not much different from the way a dog began to salivate to the sound of a bell after Ivan Pavlov, the famous Russian physiologist, paired the sound with the sight and smell of food. Just like with Pavlov's dog, the response to such foods becomes automatic. Food makers build on this knowledge. In TV advertisements, food is often paired with people having fun eating or, as in a recent burger ad, with a beautiful model in a bikini, suggesting that a particular food will make you happier or even sexier.

If you doubt that just the thought of a favorite food in which the key ingredients are fat, sugar, or salt, or some combination of them can turn on your appetite, imagine that food directly in front of your nose right now. In order to demonstrate this effect in my lectures, I would first ask if there were any folks in the audience who liked chocolate. A goodly number would raise their hands. Then I would hold up a chocolate bar for a few moments and ask them if they felt anything happening in their mouths. With looks of surprise, most of them would hold up their hands once again. They found they were salivating at the sight of the bar as if they were going to eat the chocolate. Try it out for yourself.

Of course, enterprising food manufacturers capitalize on this natural tendency and design "unnatural" foods that will turn on our appetites more than anything found in nature. Knowing the preference for fat, salt, and sweetness, scientists can design "supernormal" foods, which blend these characteristics with natural and artificial flavorings to the point that they will stimulate our appetite far beyond what we need for survival. Just about all of us have appetites that turn off before we overeat apples or other fruits, vegetables, or grains. But most of our appetites will not turn off before overeating candy bars or other confections, chips, or fried foods. Millions of dollars are spent developing and advertising such foods because if we didn't come to prefer them over apples and oranges, these food manufacturers would have a difficult time showing any profits!

Some Examples

I was told by a person in the food industry that he knew of one candy company that held focus groups with overweight women to test new chocolates to see what blend of fat, sugar, and flavorings they liked best. As a result, the company slightly increased the fat content while slightly decreasing the sugar content in one of their chocolate bars.

On May 11, 2011, *The Tennessean* carried a front-page headline, "Goo Goo Gets a Makeover." Below that headline was a picture of two Goo Goo Clusters and the notice that their ingredients had been upgraded. This news apparently deserved a headline in the Nashville paper because the Goo Goo Cluster factory is located in Nashville, and sales of the candy have been decreasing for the past thirty years.

The ingredients of the Goo Goo Cluster are chocolate, marshmallow, caramel, and nuts. However, compared with the old manufacturing process, "the new system makes for a different texture—a more aerated, lighter nougat" that is infused with the caramel, rather than adding the layer of caramel on top of the hardened nougat as done previously. The company is using a higher-grade milk chocolate and eliminating one artificial flavoring. The new version "just gets better in your mouth." One of the company executives explained that in the candy market "we're definitely fighting for space in your brain that you've reserved for a candy bar." The purpose of the new manufacturing process is to increase the palatability of the Goo Goo via a better mouthfeel and perception of the flavor complex. In all of the different versions of the Goo Goo, about 50 percent of the calories are from fat (now to be a nonhydrogenated fat—I suspect to attract the more health-conscious candy aficionados as well as to create a more tempting confection).

I was once invited to Nashville's largest food distributor on the day the company was testing desserts for the sales force. Two long tables were laid out with a selection of desserts beyond one's wildest imagination. The group circulated around the table, tasting and rating. The purpose? This was a way to give the salespeople something of the aura of a wine steward as they described the taste of the various desserts they were to encourage their clients, the city's major restaurants and groceries, to buy (and to buy from them rather than from one of the other distributors in Nashville).

One day, when I turned on my computer to begin work on this chapter, I was greeted by a pop-up window from Dunkin' Donuts advertising its new Big 'N Toasty Breakfast Sandwich (in full color of course). This breakfast sandwich contains 580 calories, 35 grams of fat, 1370 milligrams of sodium, and 1 gram of fiber. When you pair it with oven toasted hash browns, you add 200 more calories, 11 grams of fat, 730 milligrams of sodium, and 3 grams of fiber. That's a total of 780 calories, 46 grams of fat (414 fat calories), 2100 milligrams of sodium, and a measly 4 grams of fiber.

In a daily diet of 2000 calories, the U.S. government's 2010 Dietary Guidelines for Americans recommends between 20 and 35 percent of total calories in fat (400 to 700 calories), 2400 milligrams of sodium for healthy individuals (1500 milligrams for people with hypertension or diabetes, and for African-Americans), and between 25 and 35 grams of fiber daily. According to data published by the National Weight Control Registry, people who lose weight and keep it off consume 23 to 24 percent of calories in fat daily (about 46 to 47 grams of fat), which suggests that the new Big 'N Toasty Breakfast Sandwich with hash browns contains a full day's worth of fat calories for anyone wishing to maintain a weight loss.

The ingredients for the Dunkin' Donuts sandwich and hash browns are listed on the company's website and read more like a complex chemical formula than a recipe for a healthy breakfast. You might find it revealing to look up the ingredients in your favorite foods, both in the dishes in national restaurant chains and in the processed foods you buy at the supermarket. Indeed, many health-conscious people report that just reading the complete list of ingredients in processed foods has completely turned off their appetites for them. In any event, you will discover that companies making high-fat, sweet, and salty foods pay little attention to the 2010 Dietary Guidelines for Americans, which encourage us to reduce fat and sodium in our diets and to eat more whole grains, fruit, and vegetables.

One final illustration: In years gone by, I was frequently invited to lead workshops on nutrition, weight loss, and fitness. On one such occasion I was asked to present daily lectures to a group of Tennessee state government employees who were participating in a week-long retreat at an inn near one of our beautiful state parks. From Monday through Thursday, the innkeeper sent a large selection of fruit, including apples, grapes, bananas, plums, and peaches, to the meeting room during the morning break. Each day, every piece of fruit disappeared. On Friday, as a special treat, the innkeeper had the resident baker make a great batch of chocolate-chip and oatmeal-raisin cookies, which she sent along with the fruit. The group descended on the cookies with all the decorum of a pack of hungry wolves. The entire selection of cookies disappeared in minutes. One apple was eaten. The rest of the fruit was returned to the kitchen. When it comes to foods that turn on appetite, food scientists will win out over Mother Nature every time.

To succeed in permanent weight management you need to break the connection between supernormal foods and your present response to them. How can you do this? A lot occurs between the appearance of stimuli in the environment and your brain's response, which leads to your hand putting the food that gives you pleasure in your mouth. It's a long chain of events that you can learn to control. I'll describe how in Chapters 9 and 10, where I discuss how you start to include some of these foods back into your diet.

The question right now is, "How far are you willing to go in controlling your appetite for supernormal foods to achieve a quick weight loss?" My approach of cutting out *all* such foods for three weeks is still a contrarian one. The "go slow, make small changes approach" continues to be the basis of many university and commercial weight-management programs.

I am not satisfied with the weight-loss results that the go-slow-make-small-changes approaches generally achieve. Even the winner of *Consumer Reports* diet ratings (Jenny Craig at Home, June 2011 issue) achieved an average loss of 8 percent of body weight, which was maintained among participants in a two-year study. While a 5 to 10 percent loss of body weight may reduce some risk of hypertension, diabetes, and certain cancers, it adds up to about 12 pounds for a woman 25 pounds over the healthy weight of the reference woman (five feet four inches tall, 151 pounds vs. 126 pounds, see page 22 and Appendix B). For a quick weight loss that you can learn to make permanent, I think my contrarian "cut out the junk food for three weeks" is worth a serious try. Whether you use my personal cold-turkey method or the prescribed menus and recipes that were used in the WMP, there is enough flexibility in the use of *free vegetables* and *safe fruits* to never go hungry and still achieve close to a 13-pound weight loss in three weeks.

But a final word of warning: If for any reason you decide to stop following the program in one or two weeks while having lost only 5 or 10 pounds, DO NOT RETURN TO YOUR FORMER EATING HABITS before you read Chapters 9 and 10. I'll show you there how to include some supernormal foods in your diet without regaining the weight you have lost.

WINNING THE WAR

The war metaphor has been used often in describing what it takes to lose weight and keep it off. One participant in the WMP said to me, as she was struggling with her love of certain supernormal foods, that it was like different parts of her brain were at war with each other. She was right.

Your job, like hers, is to put your rational brain in command of the appetite centers that respond to food. You will need to practice new thoughts and behaviors that interrupt the old patterns that led to overeating. I will show you how to do so here and throughout the next chapters, especially Chapters 9 and 10.

Three things are required to achieve the greatest success with the Rotation Diet:

1. You need to be clear about your goal.
2. You must develop a plan of action that ensures you will reach that goal. Just having a goal of losing weight won't cut it. Your plan of action must be clear in all its behavioral details.
3. Having a winning attitude is essential. In my experience,

the most successful people aim high, even to perfection. There is one quality that successful people have that others lack: *they never give up.*

Let's talk about these three things in detail.

Your Goal

Your goal in the Rotation Diet is to stick with the particular plan you choose (cold turkey or planned menus) for three weeks. You are not going to force yourself to stick with it until any set amount of weight is lost, but you are going to commit yourself to eliminating the supernormal foods that interfere with losing weight quickly. Choose three weeks on your calendar to begin the Rotation Diet when reaching your goal will not be complicated by celebratory events, vacation, or travel. However, if something so overwhelming happens that you end up deviating from the plan you have chosen, you have only lost a skirmish. You must not permit a lapse to signal defeat. Accept your human weakness, get back on track, and aim for the very best you can do all over again. I yo-yoed for years before I found the way that worked for me. You'll find that you can learn from experience and that practice can make perfect. If you have more than 15 pounds to lose, your second twenty-one-day rotation should be even better and easier than the first.

The Detailed Plain of Action

Using the cold-turkey approach requires a different kind of planning than following the suggested recipes and menus. In Chapter

3 I gave you an idea of the foods I used and the meals I designed during the rotations on my 4S-Diet. You are going to have to do the same, planning to have the foods you prefer to eat in the home, and finding a place to eat out that serves the food that fits your plan. Using the controlled-calorie version, with its suggested recipes and menus, requires shopping ahead for the right foods, and planning to do whatever meal preparation is required. In the next chapter I will go over in more detail the preliminary arrangements you need to make as you get started. In Chapter 7 you will find the menus, recipes, a shopping list, and the rest of the information you need to follow the controlled-calorie version of the diet.

Remember: Increasing activity is a key component of the Rotation Diet. Study Chapter 8 and begin to implement the 200-calorie solution from Day 1 of the program.

The Winning Attitude

Your motivation for losing weight and your attitude about your ability to do what it takes are closely related. As I explained in Chapter 3, losing weight was a life-or-death issue for me. Weight loss has to be an important goal for you too. I can show you how to reach that goal quickly and easily, reinforcing your initial motivation, but you have to have enough motivation to put the whole plan into action. That plan must include the behaviors necessary for permanent maintenance as well as weight loss. People who have used diets in which the main strategy is the temporary elimination of supernormal foods say that the first three days are the hardest. But after that period, their motivation is reinforced by their quick weight loss, and their appetite is more easily satisfied with free vegetables and safe fruits.

Nothing reinforces a winning attitude better than, well, winning! Competitive athletes, performing musicians, and actors and actresses use fantasy, imagination, mental rehearsal, and practice in order to come as close to perfection as they can in their crafts. The techniques I employed can be very useful to you in achieving permanent weight management. I describe them in Chapter 10, which you need to read before beginning the Rotation Diet. They will help you become a winner in the weight war.

6

GETTING STARTED ON
THE RIGHT FOOT

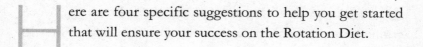ere are four specific suggestions to help you get started that will ensure your success on the Rotation Diet.

1. Take charge of your social environment. Make sure your family, friends, and coworkers know that you are about to start a three-week diet. If the people in your environment can have an impact on your behavior (and they usually can and do), you will do better with their complete cooperation.
2. Take charge of your physical environment, eliminating any hazards to your diet and adding encouragement to stay on it in your home and work office.
3. Make sure you have the exact foods you plan to eat during the Rotation Diet already available when you start the diet, and plan your menus according to the directions I give you in the next chapter. If you plan to eat any meals in restaurants during the three weeks of the Rotation Diet, you will need to follow my special recommendations for dining out. I was able to eat lunches in a restaurant five days a week, and go out to dinner occasionally, and still succeed. So can you.

4. Create a plan to increase your daily energy expenditure by 200 calories.

AVOID FOOD TRAPS AT HOME

I don't think I could have succeeded as easily as I did in losing and keeping weight off without getting complete support from my family and without setting up an inviolable time for my daily tennis match.

I announced my intentions to my wife and requested that for three weeks we not bring any foods into the house that would tempt me to eat something that was not on my plan. After all, it was only for three weeks. Everyone wanted me to succeed, so I had no problem doing this. We brought no ice cream into the house during this period, and we baked no cheesecakes, both of which happened to be among my favorite high-calorie foods at that time.

I decided to remove temptation from my house completely, right from day one, rather than try to learn to deal with my appetite and change my eating habits gradually. I needed to lose weight quickly. There was no way in the world I could fool myself into disliking my favorite foods. If they were in the house, I knew from past experience that I would ultimately end up eating them. I had no time to wait while I learned which behavior-change strategies would work and which would not when it came to resisting temptation. That could wait for the periods when I experimented with maintenance, not with weight loss.

However, when it comes to implementing the very best strategy for weight loss—*removing all temptation temporarily from your home*—you, unfortunately, may not find that your family is as cooperative as mine was, especially if you are a woman! Even for the brief three-week period that I am suggesting, you may meet with almost insurmountable resistance. You are likely to hear, from your husband and the kids, "Why do we have to go on a diet because you are trying to lose weight?" One woman in the WMP described how her overweight mate kept bringing home selections of his favorite cookies, saying to her when she objected to having them around, "You don't have to eat them." Another brought home several varieties of processed fat-free desserts, such as coffee cake and doughnuts, without realizing that these foods had been engineered to mimic the taste of the "real thing" and contained approximately the same number of calories because of their sugar content.

Responses such as these, frequently received by women when trying to make changes in their diets, make me very angry. I am amazed with how uncooperative men can be when it comes to helping the women they say they love to lose weight. In comparison with women, men with families usually have no problems when they announce they need to change their diet and get active. Everyone rallies round, out goes the junk food, Mom makes low-calorie main dishes, and everyone falls in line to take care of things when Dad goes out to exercise. When Dad makes an unequivocal statement about what he wants, most families seem ready to cooperate.

In part because of the family cooperation that men tend to receive, they find it much easier to lose weight. They also find it much easier to stay active after weight loss. If you are a woman about to begin the Rotation Diet, you need to get together with your husband and anyone else in your home and spend some time together planning how the family is going to deal with your decision. You may find everyone expects you to maintain the status quo and keep all the supernormal foods in the house that have contributed to your weight problem. Does everyone expect you to continue to prepare all of the high-fat and high-sugar dishes to which the family has been accustomed? Does everyone expect you to continue without interruption to play exactly the same roles you have played—mother and wife (possibly with a job outside the home)—and not inconvenience anyone with a change in your diet or physical activities because you would like to be healthier, happier, and more pleased with yourself?

I talked with one successful woman from the National Weight Control Registry who found it very difficult to respond to the demands for high-fat food at dinnertime. Finally she took a drastic step. One night she made the dinner she thought appropriate, put it down on the table, and, when the complaints started, announced, "That's what I have made for dinner. If you don't like it, make your own." After the uproar died down, an agreement was reached: Mom would make nutritious dinners; if Dad and the kids wanted ice cream, cake, or the like, Dad would take them out after dinner for "a treat" a few nights a week. Or he might bring home (well concealed) just enough for them to have a treat after dinner, and only bring it out after Mom had left the room.

If you are a woman, watch out, however, for something very subtle in your own attitudes about what you feed the family. As the saying goes, you may be caught "between a rock and a hard place." You, like many women, may not feel like a "good mother" or a "good wife" unless you provide your family with junk food. You may obtain a great deal of satisfaction from the joy your family derives from eating these foods. As someone who cares for her family, you may not feel that you are showing that love, or that you are, yourself, fully loved or lovable, unless you see your brood relishing supernormal foods even though they are not particularly good for their health on a daily basis. You may be equating love and caring with the food you feed the family! Watch out! If you share any of the feelings I am talking about, you need to stop and think, and realize that equating love and caring with the cookie jar does no one any good.

AVOID FOOD TRAPS OUTSIDE THE HOME

At the first meeting of a new group in the WMP we took a few minutes for participants to introduce themselves to each other and say a few words about themselves. There was no need to talk about weight. But one woman told the group that she worked in the administrative offices of the university and had gained 50 pounds in the last year. That was a conversation stopper.

Three years before joining this group she had taken leave of her job to do missionary work in sub-Saharan Africa. While living there she worked with the native women in subsistence farming and ate the local diet. None of the processed supernormal foods that surround us here in America were available. During the two years she was there, she lost 50 pounds. Now home again, working at a desk all day long and eating a supernormal American diet, she had regained all the weight she lost in Africa. When she mentioned that a popular restaurant near the university was a favorite place for lunch, part of the problem became obvious. The restaurant was famous for its steak and biscuits, served with string-cut French fries, and even more famous for its Triple Chocolate

Brownie, a fudge brownie topped with a scoop of chocolate ice cream and hot fudge sauce.

If you are likely to expose yourself to a problematic lunchtime situation similar to what I have just described, there is only one solution. You have to bring your own lunch to work or find a different restaurant where you can lock into foods that fit your plan. As I described in Chapter 3, I found that the Campus Grill near my office could serve me one of three dishes that I included in my diet. To keep away from temptation, I wouldn't even look at the menu.

If you are a woman about to begin the Rotation Diet, you will do best if you carry your own lunch and avoid eating out as much as possible. When you are in the 1200-calorie week, there are more choices in most restaurants and many frozen-food entrées in the 300-calorie range that can be stored if a freezer and a microwave are available at your workplace. Men will have little trouble finding a way to eat out or use frozen entrées since their daily calorie limit never drops below 1200.

If you are going to use my cold-turkey approach to the Rotation Diet and continue to eat out, the rule is simply to have no supernormal foods. That means no high-fat foods like a super-sized cheeseburger and no fried foods. A plain hamburger or sliced turkey sandwich with a side salad is a better choice.

If you must eat out socially, even when you are attempting to follow the prescribed meals and menus and calorie levels, think about your plan of action in advance. I have already explained how I used my "4S-Diet" label to ward off my "well-intentioned" friends who might tempt me to deviate on social occasions. When invited out to dinner at someone's home, I would always let them know in advance if I was in my "diet cycle" and would be eating lightly. For me, this meant skipping the drinks, omitting dessert (other than fruit and a piece of cheese if it was served) and bread, and scraping off any sauce if my host had chosen to prepare something that was especially rich for the main course.

I used similar strategies when dining out with friends. I was not bashful about asking whether dishes on the restaurant menu could be prepared in the least caloric way (meat, fish, or poultry grilled, with no sauce other than a bit of oil if necessary). I was surprised at the quick collaboration I received wherever we went to eat.

Remember, most people trying to lose weight often fail in a social situation because they are in conflict. Friends may encourage you to taste the dishes they have ordered (or at the end of the meal, to split a dessert "just this once"). You must make an unequivocal statement about your intentions, to yourself and to others, and stick to it. The more you make your intentions known, the more you will reinforce your commitment and ensure your success. In contrast, giving in tends to lead to giving in again.

ADDING EXERCISE TO YOUR DAY

I have a great deal of advice to give you about how to burn the 200 calories a day that is key to permanent weight management. If you are a sedentary person, I assure you that if you follow my advice to experiment with the many ways that you can add movement to your daily life, as I describe fully in Chapter 8, you will end up a slimmer and more vigorous person than you are today. So it is important that you read Chapter 8 before you begin to use the Rotation Diet.

For now, since it is frequently difficult for women who work outside the home and still fulfill all of their usual household responsibilities to find time to take a walk each day, I want to tell you how one member in the WMP solved the problem.

A schoolteacher in my group was frustrated by a work and family schedule that made it impossible to get out for a thirty- to forty-minute walk each day. She had three school-aged children and had to get up early to prepare breakfast for them and get herself ready for school. When she got home, in addition to making dinner, she had to take care of the assignments from her classes that day and make preparations for the next day's classes. She felt her husband was doing a pretty fair share of work, cleaning up after dinners and carrying out many other responsibilities around the house.

I asked her about breakfast: what does her husband do while she prepares breakfast for the kids? Her response was that he didn't need to get up quite as early as she did. I suggested that she ask her husband to consider getting the kids their breakfast while she went for an early-morning walk. He was very reluctant at first. He didn't feel competent to take on that responsibility, never having done it before. But he agreed to try after she explained precisely what it would take. Within a few days, he was very pleased with himself. He and the kids were having a good time at breakfast, and within a couple of weeks, he admitted that he was very happy with the situation. Being with the kids at breakfast had led to a much closer bond with them than ever before.

A FINAL WORD OF ADVICE

The Rotation Diet is the best quick-weight-loss plan that I know of. If you can be close to perfect, you can expect to average an enviable two-thirds of a pound of weight loss per day over the first three weeks. But I know the unexpected is to be expected. By that I mean, you may feel an almost irresistible urge to eat something not on the plan simply because someone puts it right in front of your nose and catches you off guard. There's a party at work, for example, or you find yourself dying for a little something before going to bed.

I anticipated such problems as I began my first round on my diet. Because I did not want to feel deprived, and I didn't want to listen to my stomach growling, I decided I needed to have "safe food" that I liked reasonably well and that would not do much damage to my weight-loss effort, even if I ate a lot of it. However, choosing a safe food presented me with a problem. I knew I could eat *free vegetables* to my heart's content. However, I wanted something that was more satisfying than the free vegetables, but still healthful and filling, while containing relatively few calories.

I decided that my safe food would be a fruit. Compared with other foods, fruit provides the most satisfaction in taste and bulk for the least amount of calories. And, in addition, I wanted something I liked so that it would be a reasonable substitution for foods that are much higher in calories.

I selected grapefruit. A whole grapefruit has only about 110 calories. I carried one to the office in my briefcase and made a vow that I would have to eat that grapefruit instead of any high-calorie snack that happened my way. At least, I would say to myself that

I had to eat it first, and then if I wanted to, I could eat something else. But I never did. Every time I peeled the grapefruit, I thought about how well I was losing weight, and how a high-calorie snack would slow me down. I would then break the grapefruit up into sections, and eat them, one at a time, as slowly as I could. If I was still hungry when I finished, I would drink a glass of water. I did the same at night whenever I felt hungry before going to bed.

While you are on the Rotation Diet, I don't want you to feel deprived either. However, you don't have to be as limited in your choice of *safe fruit* as I was or as the original research participants in this diet were. Since the caloric value of most fresh fruit is similar, and subsequent experience showed it didn't seem to make much difference in the amount of weight lost if participants chose more than one safe fruit, you can feel free to do the same.

I want you, too, to take a vow that safe fruit is the only extra food you will eat while you are following the plan, no matter what temptations present themselves. Keep a variety around the house. Right now, as usual, I have grapes, an apple, a grapefruit, a bunch of bananas, and several tomatoes (often considered either fruit or vegetable) prominently displayed in my kitchen.

In the next chapter, in addition to a list of *free vegetables*, I will give you a list of fresh *safe fruits*. Have plenty at home and have some to carry with you at all times. Your safe fruit is your charm, protecting you from the appetite of your former overweight self, as well as from the temptations in your environment. In just two or three days, your friends will become accustomed to seeing you dip into your bag, purse, or briefcase for your healthful snack, and they will no longer encourage you to deviate. Reaching for your safe fruit becomes a very simple thing to do. When you begin to feel a bit proud, even smug, over your ability to say, "No, thanks," to temptation as you reach for your safe fruit, you can be sure that you are securely on your way. And you can give odds to anyone silly enough to bet against your ability to end up considerably thinner in three weeks and to stay that way for good.

7

THE ROTATION DIET FOR WOMEN AND MEN

GENERAL INSTRUCTIONS

For Women

Women follow a rotation plan during Week 1 that includes approximately 600 calories a day for three days, followed by 900 calories a day for the next four days. In Week 2, you eat approximately 1200 calories a day for the entire week. In Week 3, you repeat the 600/900-calorie rotation. You can repeat the menus of Week 1 during Week 3, or if you desire more variety, you can use the Alternate Menus for the Rotation Diet in Chapter 11.

For Men

Men follow a rotation plan during Week 1 that includes approximately 1200 calories a day for three days, followed by 1500 calories a day for the next four days. In Week 2, you eat approximately 1800 calories a day for the entire week. In Week 3, you repeat the 1200/1500-calorie rotation. You can repeat the menus of Week 1 during Week 3, or if you desire more variety, you can use the Alternate Menus for the Rotation Diet in Chapter 11.

Expected Weight Loss

On average, persons who follow the Rotation Diet with few deviations will lose over 5 pounds the first week, around 2½ pounds the second week, and up to 5 pounds again the third week. The heavier you are to begin with, the more you can expect to lose, with an average of up to 1 pound a day. Despite the calorie intake for men being higher, men will tend to lose weight faster than women. Men need more calories than women to maintain their initial weight, and they burn more calories in physical activity because they tend to be heavier. In addition, heavier people tend to retain more water and will lose more water weight as they begin the reducing diet.

The use of even large quantities of *free vegetables* will do very little to detract from the expected weight loss because they contain so few calories. *Safe fruits* can add a few more calories per serving than the free vegetables. We found that women using large quantities of both may end up losing on average only ½ pound a day. Still they end up with a loss of 10½ pounds in twenty-one days. The use of both free vegetables and safe fruits will help you adhere to the plan for the full three weeks and protect you from being tempted by the high-calorie snacks and desserts that have prevented you from achieving permanent weight management in the past.

DIRECTIONS FOR USING FREE VEGETABLES

Certain foods have so few calories that you can eat them in unlimited quantities. I call them *free vegetables*. Because of their water and fiber content, relative to the number of calories they contain, it is difficult to eat enough of them to prevent yourself from losing weight, provided you follow my other suggestions exactly. Thus, whenever you see "unlimited free vegetables" on my menus, you can eat from the following list of vegetables until you feel satisfied (if you add salad dressing, use only my No-Cal Salad Dressing, page 119, or a no-calorie commercial variety).

You are also able to add free vegetables to any meal and to nibble on them as snacks. Because they contain so many vitamins and minerals (plus fiber) in relation to their caloric content, you will be increasing the nutritional value of your diet tremendously if you do so.

asparagus	chard	radishes
bamboo shoots	collard greens	spinach
broccoli	cucumber	summer squash
Brussels sprouts	green beans	tomatoes
cabbage	kale	turnip greens
carrots	lettuce	water chestnuts
cauliflower	mushrooms	wax beans
celery	onions	zucchini

DIRECTIONS FOR CHOOSING SAFE FRUITS

The *free vegetables* will let you round out your meals so that you never have to feel hungry when you have finished the prescribed lunch or dinner. But if you are at all like me, free vegetables are not always satisfying—they don't have much flavor eaten alone, and, perhaps more important, they have so few calories that they don't give you very much of a lift when you really need one. That's why I think you should choose *safe fruits* to fall back on whenever you feel hungry between meals or are tempted by some rich dessert. Although I stuck with only grapefruit while losing weight, subsequent experience with the Rotation Diet showed that participants in the WMP could use a variety of fruits with little impact on their total weight loss over the three-week diet. I think of fruits as Mother Nature's great allies, not only in a person's efforts to lose weight, but even more so when it comes to weight maintenance. The word *fruit* comes from a Latin word meaning enjoyment or to enjoy. I know that I am going to stay slim and healthy every time I substitute a piece of fruit for an enticing, but less healthful, junk-food creation!

Safe fruits do contain calories: from 40 calories for a small apple to 110 for a whole grapefruit. For this reason, they can give you a lift when you feel low on energy. The lift and the bulk provided by the water and fiber help you to stick with your diet until your next regular meal. The fruit sugar that it contains makes a safe fruit taste pretty good—not as good, perhaps, as your favorite high-calorie foods, because safe fruits don't contain any fat, but good enough to keep you from indulging. Keep reminding yourself that every time you choose safe fruits, you are avoiding a high-calorie food that will add fat to your body.

Choosing safe fruits as snacks is very important from a psychological standpoint. The choice becomes symbolic of your weight-loss effort. You carry safe fruit with you to work and make sure it's always available at home. Every time you get the urge to deviate from the Rotation Diet, you reach for it. Believe me, it's a charm! It's your absolute guarantee of success. Even if you have two or three servings a day during the 600/900-calorie rotations—a mid-morning snack, a mid-afternoon snack, a bed-time snack—you cannot add much more than 150 to 200 calories to your intake. *YOU WILL STILL LOSE WEIGHT.* It may be only 8 or 10 pounds in three weeks instead of 12 or 15, but that is a great success. And you can repeat the diet after a week off and lose more weight. (Safe fruits are built into the diet at levels of 1200 calories and above, without exceeding calorie limits.)

apples	oranges
berries	peaches
grapefruit	pears
grapes	pineapple
melons	tangerines

Warning: Grapefruit is known to interact with certain drugs. If you are on any prescription medications, check with your physician about the advisability of including grapefruit or grapefruit juice in your diet.

BEVERAGES

Although nutritionists no longer feel it necessary to recommend that people drink eight glasses of water a day, water remains the drink of choice. I think most people who have stopped using water as the main source of liquid in their diets have found that water right out of the faucet doesn't taste particularly good. In addition, there can be the smell of chlorine. To make your water taste better, get a home filter for your faucet, or use a pitcher with a filter, and add a slice of lemon or lime. You should limit yourself to two cups of tea or coffee (black preferred, but a teaspoon of half-and-half will add only 8 calories). Too much caffeine can make some people jittery while they are cutting calories. Herb teas are good in moderation, but avoid those with laxative qualities. Try low-salt bouillons for a change (or make your own stock with meat, chicken, or vegetables; see one of my recipes on page 112).

FOOD PREPARATION AND SIZE OF SERVINGS

Prepare your food simply. Add no fat during the 600-calorie rotation, and use only the very small amounts of fat prescribed during the 900- and 1200-calorie rotations. Learn to use herbs and spices in place of salt (see discussion of salt below).

I have developed recipes to illustrate delicious ways of preparing foods with few added fat calories. Items in the Rotation Diet plan menus that have recipes in this book are followed by an asterisk. (Recipes for the basic Rotation Diet begin on page 101.)

The correct serving sizes in either weight or volume are given both with the menus and with my recipes, and the approximate number of calories in each serving is given with the recipes. If you do not have a good idea of serving sizes, it is worth buying a scale and other measuring implements and weighing the amounts for a few days. Then you will have portion sizes stored in your memory, and you can discontinue the practice.

However, if you dislike weighing, measuring, and counting calories as much as I do, then, for convenience, all you need to remember when you prepare foods your own way, or when eating out, is that you will tend to be within the dietary guidelines when you choose standard, or moderate cafeteria-sized portions, not the supersized portions advertised at many fast-food restaurants.

Here is a rough guide to help estimate portion sizes:

- 1 fist = 1 cup of cereal, pasta, or vegetables
- 1 finger = 1 ounce of cheese
- 1 thumb tip = 1 teaspoon of peanut butter, butter, or sugar
- 1 palm = 3 ounces of fish, or poultry
- 1 deck of cards = 3 ounces of cooked meat
- 1 handful = 1 ounce of chips, nuts, or pretzels
- 1 tennis ball = 1 medium fruit serving
- 1 Ping-Pong ball = 2 tablespoons of butter, peanut butter, or salad dressing

Standard Portions for Vegetables

Generally, a standard portion for vegetables (other than *free vegetables*) is a ½ cup. Some vegetables have so few calories that standard portions are as large as 1 cup. You will see which vegetables fall into each category as you follow the diet. And, of course, many vegetables are unlimited in the amount you can have (see list on page 375 or 385).

Standard Portions for Meat, Fish, and Fowl

For meat, fish, and fowl, a standard portion to fit the Rotation Diet plans for women during the 600/900-calorie rotations is generally 3 ounces cooked weight (about 4 ounces raw). (Exceptions are noted in the daily menus.) Portions for women go up to either 4½ ounces or 6 ounces cooked (about 6 to 8 ounces raw) during the 1200-calorie rotation.

Portions for men are either 4½ or 6 ounces cooked weight (6 to 8 ounces raw) during the 1200-calorie rotations, and 6 ounces cooked (about 8 ounces raw) during the 1500- and 1800-calorie rotations. Note: The variation in the recommended portions depends in part on what is on the rest of the day's menu, and the calories in the meat or fish itself.

Standard Portions for Grain Foods

1 slice of bread
1 ounce of dry cereal
½ cup of rice
1 cup pasta (cooked)
5 whole-wheat crackers

Standard Portions for Dairy Products

8 ounces of low-fat milk
8 ounces of plain non-fat or low-fat yogurt
1 ounce of hard cheese
½ cup of low-fat cottage cheese

SNACKS

During the 600/900-calorie rotations, women should stick with *free vegetables* and *safe fruits* as snacks to prevent a serious slowdown in weight loss. You may have a slight lowering of weight loss depending on how much of these vegetables and fruits you eat; however, it will be negligible compared to eating foods not on these lists. Remember, free vegetables and safe fruits are an insurance policy. Use them to help *guarantee* your weight loss.

While safe fruits are optional on all 600/900-calorie days, they are included as snacks in all menus of 1200 calories and higher. It is not obligatory for you to eat all of these snacks. When you are on a rotation with 1200 calories or more, you should experiment with having one at mid-morning, at mid-afternoon, and at bedtime. As I indicated, I never went to bed hungry. And after a grapefruit snack at bedtime, I always slept well, without waking up famished in the middle of the night.

SUBSTITUTIONS

Even on the 600/900-calorie days, the meals have been designed to supply, insofar as possible, the Recommended Dietary Allowances (RDAs) of the major vitamins and minerals, and to preserve your electrolyte balance, which affects heart rhythm. There is more flexibility during the 1200-calorie rotation, although you should make substitutions in accordance with certain dietary principles, which I discuss later in this chapter. Both men and women can have great flexibility when they reach 1500 calories. If you need to make substitutions in any of the menus, whether because of lack of availability or for matters of taste, please read the section on making substitutions, which begins on page 148.

AN IMPORTANT WORD ABOUT SALT

The use of salt will impede your weight loss. Either use no salt at all in food preparation or, as I suggest in my recipes, add only the smallest amount, to taste. Many persons find they can cut back on salt considerably if they do not add it until after their food is cooked. Soy sauce is also somewhat high in sodium (about one-seventh the concentration of salt granules, or about 285 milligrams per teaspoon, compared with 2000 to 2200 milligrams for salt). Therefore, do not exceed the amounts called for when I suggest the use of soy sauce in my recipes. Also look for reduced-sodium soy sauce, which is widely available.

If you generally use salt, by all means try my recipe for Herb Salt (page 147). It has one-seventh the amount of sodium in plain salt, which means that it has far less sodium in it than many commercially blended salt substitutes. Whereas just ⅛ teaspoon of salt has between 250 and 275 milligrams of sodium, Herb Salt has about 40 milligrams. Herb Salt is safer to use than soy sauce if you are serious about reducing the sodium in your diet, because you will tend to use much less of it. (Some salt substitutes completely replace the sodium component with potassium, but they tend not to taste as good as Herb Salt.)

Commercially prepared soup, such as mushroom and chicken, may contain nearly 1000 milligrams of sodium—in *one cup!* Ditto for a single serving of a frozen diet-dinner main course. As with a pickle, that much sodium can lead to pounds of water retention.

Also, since my menus often call for crackers, look for the low-salt or no-salt varieties (see page 105 for suggestions).

Many packagers of foods (canned and frozen) have lately taken note of the new low-salt consciousness and produce many "no salt added" products. I strongly suggest you try some of these.

Losing weight and getting active forty-eight years ago cured my hypertension. And I thought I still had it under control until a visit to my physician suggested otherwise. I have a familial disposition to hypertension, which has shown itself among my relatives, the majority of whom have died of stroke.

When my physician saw that my blood pressure was 180/100, he recommended that I begin immediately on hydrochlorothiazide, and was very doubtful when I suggested I try lowering my sodium intake to 1500 milligrams a day before starting on any drugs. His experience with dietary control of hypertension had not been particularly good, and among the doubtful things he said was, "You'll never be able to eat out!" But I convinced him that I had both the nutritional knowledge and the determination to actually cut my sodium intake far enough to not need drugs.

We agreed on a three-week dietary trial. I was to take my blood pressure twice a day, with a goal of 95 percent of the readings showing the systolic pressure (first number) below 130. Rather than spend time I didn't have then on developing special low- or no-salt dishes, I went straight to the supermarket and bought every Mrs. Dash no-salt seasoning on the shelf so that I could start my low-sodium diet immediately. Within three days there was a clear downward trend in my daily blood pressure readings, and by the end of the week *all* of my readings at home were below 130/80. The last time I visited my physician, my blood pressure at the office was 120/80.

Note: If you are already on blood-pressure medication and eating the typical American diet that contains 3500 milligrams or more of sodium a day, you must consult your physician before you undertake cutting your sodium intake down to 1500 milligrams. I suspect he or she will want to monitor your blood pressure and possibly adjust your medication.

THE COUPLES ROTATION DIET

While there are separate menus for women and men, couples can use the Rotation Diet together. To do this, men use the basic Rotation Diet for women and add approximately 600 calories each day, throughout the twenty-one days.

Weeks 1 and 3

For best results, in Weeks 1 and 3 men use the Rotation Diet for women and add the following daily:

2 more grain servings
50 percent larger portions of meat, fish, or fowl
1 tablespoon of butter, oil, or regular salad dressing
3 safe fruits

These are healthy choices that will make up the caloric difference and keep your meals balanced.

Week 2

In Week 2, when women are on the 1200-calorie menu and men on 1800 calories, men have a tremendous amount of flexibility. Since the 1200-calorie diet for women has been designed to provide the RDAs of essential vitamins and minerals, a man could add 600 calories to the Rotation Diet for women in many different ways and still end up with a nutritious diet. For best results during Week 2, men should use the menu for women (which already includes three safe fruits and 1 tablespoon of fat as a spread or for seasoning) and add all of the following each day:

2 more grain servings
50 percent larger portions of vegetables and main dishes

Adapting the women's diet to a male equivalent leads to about a 100-calorie disparity because the male diet for Week 2 allows for slightly more fat. However, that is the only real difference. The primary goal in designing the menus for the Rotation Diet was to meet the nutrient balance recommended by the U.S. Department of Agriculture and the Food and Drug Administration in Week 2, and to come as close as possible in Weeks 1 and 3. It is actually best to think in weekly terms about the nutritional value of your diet rather than in daily terms. I'll explain the rationale for this statement when I talk about customizing the Rotation Diet to meet food preferences for yourself and your family, below and later in this chapter on pages 148–51.

ADVICE FOR SINGLES

I know it is hard for single persons to cook nutritiously for themselves—perhaps even harder when one is on a reducing diet. Every time my wife traveled and I was alone at home for days or weeks at a time, I found myself not wishing to cook well-rounded meals. But it can be done, and done easily, with just a little planning.

The best way, I think, is to cook up servings for two (cut recipes for four in half) and refrigerate or freeze the unused portions. You will be using the same foods again later in the diet, so you will already have them on hand. Most foods will keep well for three to five days in the refrigerator, and for months in the freezer. Cover your extra serving appropriately for the refrigerator, and with freezer wrap for the freezer. You can also make the recipe for four and then freeze the food in separate, serving-size packages. That will save you time and bother in the future. My wife and I do a good deal of this large-batch cooking on weekends, and the leftovers serve us well during the coming week.

FOR THE DIETER WITH A FAMILY

If you are the only dieter in the household, use the basic menu in large enough amounts to feed everyone, adding any fattening seasonings later and separately for the rest of the family. This may not work at first because many members of the family may not be accustomed to eating a nutritious diet! They may want different foods, turn up their noses at the vegetables, and insist on fried dishes or other foods not on the diet that have lots of added fat or sugar. A microwave oven is a great gift on these occasions, since you can make your own vegetables in a couple of minutes. You may have to prepare your own menu separately—the plain-cooking style of the Rotation Diet makes it easier than if you try to follow elaborate methods of food preparation.

But if you plan in advance, you can reconcile the way you need to eat to lose weight quickly with the way your family likes their food prepared. Take a look at the menus, and see if you can make a sauce or gravy to put out for the rest of the family. And it can be a great help to make your meals in advance during the weekend. Separately freeze family-sized portions to pull out when you need them.

Remember my advice to sit down before you begin the Rotation Diet and figure out what it will take for you to approach perfection, given your particular life situation. If you talk it over with your family, explaining exactly what you need to do for the next three weeks, you can get their help and cooperation. Lay the menus for the Rotation Diet before them, and discuss what it will take to keep everybody happy as you lose weight. Please refer to pages 148–51 for more suggestions on how to customize the Rotation Diet.

COPY (OR CUT OUT) YOUR PERSONAL POCKET EDITION OF THE ROTATION DIET

For your convenience in following the Rotation Diet, I have designed a Pocket Edition of the menus that I am about to give you. The Pocket Edition for women will be found beginning on page 367, and the one for men on page 377. You can photocopy the Pocket Edition and carry it with you to help you select your foods throughout each day. You can show it to your friends when they begin to marvel at your weight loss (but if your friends decide to go on the Rotation Diet with you, make sure they follow the instructions in the Pocket Edition). In case a photocopier is not easily available to you, the pages of the Pocket Edition are arranged so that you can cut them out of the book without damaging the other contents.

THE COMPLETE ROTATION DIET PLAN
MENUS FOR WOMEN

Additional information on serving sizes, *with caloric values*, will be found with the recipes that accompany all items followed by an asterisk. Do check out these excellent recipes. They illustrate that low-calorie cooking does not have to lead to boredom and deprivation.

WEEK 1

In the case of couples who wish to use the Rotation Diet together, men may use the basic diet plan for women with the addition of all of the following each day:

2 more grain servings (bread, cereal, or crackers)
50 percent larger portions of meat, fish, or fowl
1 tablespoon of butter, oil, or regular salad dressing
3 safe fruits

The calorie goal for men is 1200 calories for the first three days, and 1500 calories for the next four.

Day 1

Breakfast ½ grapefruit, 1 slice of whole-wheat bread and 1 slice of cheese (1 ounce, see Mexican Cheese Toast*), no-cal beverage

Lunch 1 scoop of salmon (2 ounces canned in water, see Salmon with Herbs*), unlimited free vegetables, 5 whole-wheat crackers, no-cal beverage

| Dinner | Baked Chicken* (3 ounces cooked), 1 serving each of cauliflower* (1 cup) and beets* (½ cup), 1 apple, no-cal beverage |

Day 2

Breakfast	½ banana, 1 ounce of high-fiber cereal (see page 106), 8 ounces of skim or low-fat milk, no-cal beverage
Lunch	1 scoop of low-fat cottage cheese (4 ounces, see Cottage Cheese Plus*), unlimited free vegetables, 1 slice of whole-wheat bread, no-cal beverage
Dinner	Poached Fish Fillet* (3 ounces, cooked), 1 serving each of broccoli* (1 cup) and carrots* (½ cup), ½ grapefruit, no-cal beverage

Day 3

Breakfast	1 slice of whole-wheat bread, 1 tablespoon of peanut butter, 1 apple, no-cal beverage
Lunch	Luncheon Tuna Vinaigrette* (2 ounces packed in water or 3 medium sardines from Sardines Vinaigrette*), 5 whole-wheat crackers, unlimited free vegetables, no-cal beverage
Dinner	beefsteak or hamburger patty (3 ounces cooked, see Steak and Hamburger Teriyaki Style*), 1 cup of asparagus,* 1 cup of Dinner Salad,* No-Cal Salad Dressing,* 1 slice of cheese (1 ounce), 1 orange, no-cal beverage

Day 4

| Breakfast | ½ banana, 1 ounce of high-fiber cereal (see page 106), 8 ounces of skim or low-fat milk, no-cal beverage |

Lunch   Tuna Salad* (with 2 ounces of water-packed tuna), unlimited free vegetables, 2 slices of whole-wheat bread, 1 teaspoon of mayonnaise or Lo-Cal Salad Dressing,* ½ grapefruit, no-cal beverage

Dinner   Baked Chicken* (3 ounces cooked), ½ cup of carrots,* 1 cup of Dinner Salad,* 1 slice of cheese (1 ounce), 1 apple, no-cal beverage

Day 5

Breakfast   1 cup of berries, 1 serving of low-fat cottage cheese (4 ounces, see Cottage Cheese Plus*), 5 whole-wheat crackers, no-cal beverage

Lunch   Sardines Vinaigrette* (3 medium; or Luncheon Tuna Vinaigrette,* 2 ounces canned in water), unlimited free vegetables, 2 slices of whole-wheat bread, 1 teaspoon of mayonnaise or Lo-Cal Salad Dressing,* ½ grapefruit, no-cal beverage

Dinner   beefsteak or hamburger patty (3 ounces cooked, see Steak and Hamburger Teriyaki Style*), 1 serving each of green beans* (½ cup) and broccoli* (1 cup), 1 slice of cheese (1 ounce), 1 apple, no-cal beverage

Day 6

Breakfast   ½ cantaloupe, 1 slice of cheese (1 ounce) and 1 slice of whole-wheat bread (see Mexican Cheese Toast*), no-cal beverage

Lunch   1 hard-boiled egg (see Curried Unstuffed Hard-boiled Egg*), unlimited free vegetables, 2 slices of whole-wheat bread, 1 teaspoon of mayonnaise or Lo-Cal Salad Dressing,* ½ grapefruit, no-cal beverage

| Dinner | Poached (or Baked) Fish Fillet* (3 ounces), 1 serving each of asparagus* (1 cup) and green peas* (½ cup), 1 apple, no-cal beverage |

Day 7

Breakfast	½ banana, 1 ounce of high-fiber cereal (see page 106), 8 ounces of skim or low-fat milk, no-cal beverage
Lunch	1 cup of berries, 1 serving of low-fat cottage cheese (4 ounces, see Cottage Cheese Plus*), 2 slices of whole-wheat bread, no-cal beverage
Dinner	Baked Chicken* (3 ounces cooked), 1 serving each of cauliflower* (1 cup) and carrots* (½ cup), 1 apple, no-cal beverage

WEEK 2

In Week 2 women may add a mid-morning, a mid-afternoon, and an evening snack, intentionally incorporating three servings of your *safe fruit*. It is not obligatory to include all of these snacks in addition to the menus below, but they are permitted within the 1200-calorie limit for this week. You may also add 1 tablespoon of butter, margarine, oil, or regular salad dressing to your diet each day. Use it for cooking or as a spread.

For couples' use, men should add all of the following each day to the daily menus of the Rotation Diet for women, below.

2 more grain servings (bread, cereal, or crackers)
50 percent larger portions of vegetables and main courses

Optional for men: another tablespoon of fat for spread or seasoning. The calorie goal for males is 1800 per day throughout

Week 2. Additional information on serving sizes, *with caloric values*, will be found with the recipes.

Day 8

Breakfast   ½ grapefruit, 1 slice of whole-wheat bread, 1 table-spoon of peanut butter, 8 ounces of skim or low-fat milk, no-cal beverage

Lunch   large fruit salad (about 2 cups, see Creative Fruit Salad*), 1 slice of cheese (1 ounce), 5 whole-wheat crackers, no-cal beverage

Dinner   salmon steak (4½ ounces, see Royal Indian Salmon*), 1 serving of Peas and Baby Onions* (½ cup), 1 cup of Dinner Salad,* no-cal beverage

Day 9

Breakfast   ½ banana, 1 ounce of high-fiber cereal (see page 106), 8 ounces of skim or low-fat milk, no-cal beverage

Lunch   large chef salad (1 ounce each of cheese and turkey plus any salad vegetables, see Creative Chef Salad*), 5 whole-wheat crackers, Lo-Cal Salad Dressing,* no-cal beverage

Dinner   chicken (4½ ounces cooked, see Chicken Tomasi* for something special tonight), 1 small baked potato (3½ ounces), green beans (1 cup, or try Green Beans Almondine*), 1 slice of cheese (1 ounce), 1 apple, no-cal beverage

Day 10

Breakfast   sliced fresh fruit of your choice (1 cup), 1 serving of low-fat cottage cheese (4 ounces), 1 slice of whole-wheat bread, no-cal beverage

Lunch	sandwich (2 ounces of meat or cheese, or see Combination Sandwich*), unlimited free vegetables, 1 orange, no-cal beverage
Dinner	Stir-Fry Vegetables* (2 cups), Brown or Wild Rice* (½ cup), 2 tablespoons of grated cheese, 1 apple, no-cal beverage

Day 11

Breakfast	1 cup of fresh pineapple (or other fresh fruit), 1 slice of cheese (1 ounce), 1 slice of whole-wheat bread, no-cal beverage
Lunch	Spinach Salad* (large, 2–3 cups, with sliced mushrooms, green peppers, and chopped egg), Lo-Cal Salad Dressing,* 1 apple or pear, 1 slice of cheese (1 ounce), no-cal beverage
Dinner	steak (6 ounces, see Steak Flamed in Brandy* or Marinated Flank Steak*), 1 small baked potato (3½ ounces), Braised Carrots and Celery* (1 cup), ½ grapefruit, no-cal beverage

Day 12

Breakfast	sliced fruit (½ cup), 1 ounce of high-fiber cereal (see page 106), 8 ounces of skim or low-fat milk, no-cal beverage
Lunch	Tuna Salad* or Sardines Vinaigrette* (with 3 ounces of water-packed tuna or 4–5 medium sardines), unlimited free vegetables plus sliced tomato and green pepper, Lo-Cal Salad Dressing,* 1 slice of whole-wheat bread, no-cal beverage
Dinner	Herbed Pork* (6 ounces), ½ baked Acorn Squash,*

Broccoli with Black Olives* (1 cup of broccoli), ½ grapefruit, no-cal beverage

Day 13

Breakfast ½ melon, 1 hard- or soft-boiled egg, 1 slice of whole-wheat bread, no-cal beverage

Lunch dieter's special: ground-beef patty (4½ ounces cooked), 1 serving of low-fat cottage cheese (4 ounces), sliced tomato and unlimited free vegetables, Lo-Cal Salad Dressing,* no-cal beverage

Dinner My Favorite Pasta* (1 cup, plus choice of sauce), 2 tablespoons of Parmesan cheese, 1 cup of Dinner Salad,* choice of 1 fresh fruit, no-cal beverage

Day 14

Breakfast ½ grapefruit, 1 cup of oatmeal, 2 tablespoons of raisins, dash of cinnamon, 4 ounces of skim or low-fat milk, no-cal beverage

Lunch toasted open-faced sandwich (try Mexican Bean Spread,* 1 slice of cheese, and sliced tomato, or see Day 10 for a regular sandwich), unlimited free vegetables, 1 cup of assorted sliced fresh fruit, no-cal beverage

Dinner Pot Roast of Beef* (4 ounces of meat, cooked, including vegetables), 1 cup of Dinner Salad,* Lo-Cal Salad Dressing,* 1 slice of cheese (1 ounce), 1 apple, no-cal beverage

WEEK 3

Repeat the menus of Week 1, or use the Alternate Menus in Chapter 11 for the 600- and 900-calorie rotations.

When you finish your twenty-one days on the Rotation Diet, BE VERY SURE THAT YOU FOLLOW MY DIRECTIONS FOR MAKING A TRANSITION TO MAINTENANCE IN WEEK 4 (CHAPTER 9).

THE COMPLETE ROTATION DIET PLAN MENUS FOR MEN

WEEK 1

Men may incorporate three *safe fruit* snacks each day within calorie guidelines thoughout the Rotation Diet, but it is not obligatory. You may also add 1 tablespoon of butter, margarine, or regular salad dressing (in place of lo-cal) to each day's menu and remain within the calorie limits.

Day 1

Breakfast   ½ banana, 1 ounce of high-fiber cereal (see page 106), 8 ounces of skim or low-fat milk, no-cal beverage

Lunch   large chef salad (1 ounce each of cheese and turkey, plus any salad vegetables, see Creative Chef Salad*), Lo-Cal Salad Dressing,* 5 whole-wheat crackers, no-cal beverage

Dinner   Baked Chicken* (4½ ounces cooked), 1 small baked

potato (3½ o...
1 apple, 1 sli...

Day 2

Breakfast   ½ grapefrui...
spoon of pe...
milk, no-cal...

Lunch   large fruit s...
Salad*), 1 sl...
crackers, no-...

Dinner   Poached (or Baked) Fish Fillet* (6 ounces cooked),
1 serving of Peas and Baby Onions* (½ cup), Dinner Salad* (1 cup), Lo-Cal Salad Dressing,* no-cal
beverage

Day 3

Breakfast   1 cup of sliced fruit (your choice), 1 serving of low-
fat cottage cheese (4 ounces), 1 slice of whole-wheat
bread, no-cal beverage

Lunch   Combination Sandwich* (2 ounces of meat or cheese),
unlimited free vegetables, 1 orange, no-cal beverage

Dinner   Stir-Fry Vegetables* (2 cups), Brown or Wild Rice*
(½ cup), 2 tablespoons of grated cheese, 1 apple, no-
cal beverage

Day 4

Breakfast   1 cup of berries, 1½ ounces of high-fiber cereal (see
page 106), 8 ounces of skim or low-fat milk, 1 slice of
whole-wheat bread, 1 teaspoon of preserves, no-cal
beverage

Lunch   Spinach Salad* (large, 2–3 cups, with sliced mush-

Handwritten note:

Menu For men
- Years ago (30) I Lost 30 pounds in 3 weeks on this. Since then I follow it for about 4 ors Days to get back on track. I eat a Lot of Free veggies + fruits Every Day. I had to Change my Life. I Find this easy to follow

rooms, green peppers, chopped egg, and Lo-Cal Salad Dressing*), 5 whole-wheat crackers, 1 apple or pear, no-cal beverage

Dinner ½ grapefruit, steak (6 ounces cooked, see Steak Flamed in Brandy* or Marinated Flank Steak*), 1 small baked potato (3½ ounces), Braised Carrots and Celery* (1 cup), no-cal beverage

Day 5

Breakfast ½ melon, 1 hard- or soft-boiled egg, 2 slices of whole-wheat bread, 1 teaspoon of preserves, no-cal beverage

Lunch ground-beef patty (4½ ounces cooked, see Steak and Hamburger Teriyaki Style*), 1 serving of low-fat cottage cheese (4 ounces), unlimited free vegetables, 1 slice of whole-wheat bread, 1 serving of fruit (your choice), no-cal beverage

Dinner My Favorite Pasta* (1 cup, plus choice of sauce), 4 tablespoons of grated Parmesan cheese, Dinner Salad* (1 cup), Lo-Cal Salad Dressing,* ½ grapefruit, no-cal beverage

Day 6

Breakfast 1 cup of sliced fruit, 1½ ounces of high-fiber cereal (see page 106), 1 slice of whole-wheat bread, 8 ounces of skim or low-fat milk, no-cal beverage

Lunch Tuna Salad* or Sardines Vinaigrette* (3 ounces of water-packed tuna, or 4–5 medium sardines), unlimited free vegetables plus sliced tomato and green pepper, Lo-Cal Salad Dressing,* 2 slices of whole-wheat bread, no-cal beverage

Dinner   Herbed Pork* (6 ounces cooked), ½ baked Acorn Squash,* Broccoli with Black Olives* (1 cup of broccoli), 1 slice of whole-wheat bread, ½ grapefruit, no-cal beverage

Day 7

Breakfast ½ grapefruit, 1 cup of oatmeal, 2 tablespoons of raisins, dash of cinnamon, 4 ounces of skim or low-fat milk, no-cal beverage

Lunch   open-faced sandwich (2 portions, see Mexican Bean Spread,* with 1 slice of cheese and sliced tomato, or see Day 3 for a regular sandwich), unlimited free vegetables, Lo-Cal Salad Dressing,* 1 cup of assorted fresh fruit, no-cal beverage

Dinner   Pot Roast of Beef* (4 ounces of meat, including vegetables), Dinner Salad* (1 cup), Lo-Cal Salad Dressing,* 1 apple, no-cal beverage

WEEK 2

During Week 2 you can add 1 tablespoon of butter, margarine, or regular salad dressing to each day's menu, as well as the three *safe fruits*, and remain within the calorie limits.

Day 8

Breakfast ½ melon, 2 slices of whole-wheat bread, 2 slices of cheese (2 ounces), no-cal beverage

Lunch   Tuna-Salad Sandwich* (3 ounces of water-packed tuna), unlimited free vegetables, 1 serving of fruit (your choice), no-cal beverage

Dinner   Baked Chicken* (6 ounces cooked), Spinach and

Broccoli Casserole* (½ cup, or 1 cup of broccoli plainly prepared), ½ baked Acorn Squash,* 1 apple, 1 slice of cheese (1 ounce; if casserole recipe is not used), no-cal beverage

Day 9

Breakfast   1 cup of oatmeal, 2 tablespoons of raisins, dash of cinnamon, 4 ounces of skim or low-fat milk, 1 slice of whole-wheat bread, 1 teaspoon of preserves, no-cal beverage

Lunch   large fruit salad (2 cups, see Creative Fruit Salad*), 1 serving of low-fat cottage cheese (4 ounces), 5 whole-wheat crackers, no-cal beverage

Dinner   Baked (or Poached) Fish Fillet* (6 ounces), Baked Tomato* (½ tomato), 1 small baked potato (3½ ounces), Dinner Salad* (1 cup), 1 slice of cheese (1 ounce), 1 apple, no-cal beverage

Day 10

Breakfast   1 orange, 2 slices of whole-wheat bread, 2 slices of cheese (2 ounces), no-cal beverage

Lunch   Tuna Salad* (3 ounces of water-packed tuna) on greens with sliced tomatoes and green pepper, plus unlimited free vegetables, Lo-Cal Salad Dressing,* no-cal beverage

Dinner   steak (6 ounces cooked, see Marinated Flank Steak* or Steak Flamed in Brandy*), Stir-Fry Spinach* (1 cup), 1 small baked potato (3½ ounces) with Cottage-Cheese Dressing* (or 2 tablespoons of sour cream), choice of 1 fruit, no-cal beverage

Day 11

Breakfast   ½ melon, 1 serving of low-fat cottage cheese (4 ounces), 1 slice of whole-wheat bread, 1 teaspoon of preserves, no-cal beverage

Lunch   sandwich (2 ounces of meat or cheese, see Combination Sandwich*), unlimited free vegetables, Lo-Cal Salad Dressing,* no-cal beverage

Dinner   baked salmon (6 ounces cooked, see Royal Indian Salmon*), Peas and Baby Onions* (½ cup), Dinner Salad* (1 cup), Lo-Cal Salad Dressing,* choice of 1 fruit, 1 slice of cheese (1 ounce), no-cal beverage

Day 12

Breakfast   ½ grapefruit, 2 slices of whole-wheat bread, 1 tablespoon of peanut butter, 1 teaspoon of preserves, no-cal beverage

Lunch   1 cup of soup (commercial or see Soups*), 10 whole-wheat crackers, 2 slices of cheese (2 ounces), unlimited free vegetables, Lo-Cal Salad Dressing,* no-cal beverage

Dinner   Eggplant Casserole* (or 6 ounces, cooked, of lean meat of your choice), carrots* (½ cup), Dinner Salad* (1 cup), Lo-Cal Salad Dressing,* 1 apple, no-cal beverage

Day 13

Breakfast   1 cup of berries, 1½ ounces of high-fiber cereal (see page 106), 1 slice of whole-wheat bread, 1 teaspoon of preserves, 8 ounces of skim or low-fat milk, no-cal beverage

Lunch	large chef salad (1 ounce each of cheese and turkey, plus any salad vegetables, see Creative Chef Salad*), Lo-Cal Salad Dressing,* 5 whole-wheat crackers, no-cal beverage
Dinner	Baked Chicken* (6 ounces cooked, or try Almond Chicken*), 1 serving of Brown or Wild Rice* (½ cup), broccoli* (1 cup), 1 slice of cheese (1 ounce), 1 apple, no-cal beverage

Day 14

Breakfast	choice of sliced fruit (1 cup), 1 serving of low-fat cottage cheese (4 ounces), 1 slice of whole-wheat bread, 1 teaspoon of preserves, no-cal beverage
Lunch	sandwich (2 ounces of meat or cheese, see Combination Sandwich*), unlimited free vegetables, Lo-Cal Salad Dressing,* ½ grapefruit, no-cal beverage
Dinner	fish of your choice (6 ounces cooked, or try Baked or Broiled Rainbow Trout*), Baked Tomato* (½ tomato), Green Beans with Chives* (1 cup, or use mushroom variation), 1 slice of whole-wheat bread, 1 slice of cheese (1 ounce), 1 fruit of your choice, no-cal beverage

WEEK 3

Repeat the menus of Week 1, or use the Alternate Menus in Chapter 11 for the 1200- and 1500-calorie rotations.

When you finish your twenty-one days on the Rotation Diet, BE VERY SURE THAT YOU FOLLOW MY DIRECTIONS FOR MAKING A TRANSITION TO MAINTENANCE IN WEEK 4 (CHAPTER 9).

RECIPES

The recipes and serving suggestions for the Rotation Diet are meant to illustrate that low-calorie cooking need not be boring and without taste. However, for simplicity's sake, you may prepare everything plain, or according to your own favorite recipes, provided you do not add fat, sugar, or anything else that will increase the calorie content appreciably.

To facilitate weight loss, do not use salt. However, if you must have a small amount of salt for flavoring, it is best to add it after cooking, at the table.

See my recipe for Herb Salt (page 147), which cuts out over 85 percent of the sodium. It's a great blend.

Except for *free vegetables*, be sure to adhere to the serving sizes recommended. And, of course, remember that you have a *safe fruit* that you can use to make sure you do not feel hungry.

Grains, Breads, Crackers, Cereals

I advise you to use either 100 percent whole-grain breads and crackers or breads and crackers that have as their primary ingredient a whole grain. If the primary ingredient is a whole grain, it will be listed first on the label of a commercial product.

Breads and crackers in the grocery store that say "100 percent whole wheat" and those listing only "whole-wheat flour" as the grain ingredient will be made entirely of whole grains. Blends will list other grains or types of flour.

I like breads made from whole-grain products because they offer a wider array of vitamins and minerals than the refined-grain products and three or more times the dietary fiber.

Most commercial whole-wheat breads contain about 65 to 70 calories per slice, and the usual whole-wheat cracker has about 17 calories (five whole-wheat crackers will be about 85 calories).

BREADS

Here are two outstanding whole-wheat breads that were developed especially for the Rotation Diet by one of Nashville's outstanding bakers and teachers of baking, Ms. Joyce Weingartner. As you will see when you try these recipes, blending a small amount of other flours with the primary whole-wheat flour provides a lighter, more attractive texture than can be obtained by using only whole-wheat flour. In addition, the use of other flours in small amounts increases the overall nutritional value of the bread, since the other flours have a different array of nutrients. Both of these breads are batter breads, which makes for quick and easy baking.

WHOLE-WHEAT BATTER BREAD

In a large mixing bowl combine:

5   cups of whole-wheat flour

½   cup of barley flour (white can be substituted)

½   cup of soy flour

½   cup of sugar (you may mix ¼ cup of white and ¼ cup of brown)

1   tablespoon of salt (or just 2 teaspoons of salt, which we like, since it yields a slightly sweeter-tasting bread)

2   packages of dry yeast

Pour in 3½ cups of hot water and stir 200 strong strokes until blended.

Mixing the ingredients should take at least 3 minutes until the flours are completely incorporated. This will yield a soft batter that is not to be kneaded.

With a wooden spoon, fill two 5- by 9-inch bread pans, which have been well greased. Push dough into the corners and smooth the top surface. A wet spoon helps this process.

Cover with a warm, wet towel and place in a draft-free area until the batter has doubled.

Preheat oven to 400 degrees and bake for 15 minutes.

Reduce heat to 350 degrees and continue baking for another 45 minutes.

To prevent the top of the bread from becoming too dark, you may cover it with foil for the last half-hour of baking.

Test each loaf for a hollow sound when you remove it from the oven and the pan. If the bread is soft on the bottom, return to pans and place in the oven for about 10 additional minutes.

Remove bread from pans and place on a metal rack to cool, with a cloth over the bread.

Cool before serving.

Store in a plastic bag in the refrigerator if you plan to use it immediately (in a week, for example), or in a plastic bag in the freezer for longer periods.

Note: If you wish to have a bread that is 100 percent whole wheat, delete the barley and soy flours and use 6 cups of whole-wheat flour in this recipe.

OATMEAL BATTER BREAD

While proofing 2 packages of yeast in ¼ cup of water to which have been added ¼ teaspoon of sugar and ¼ teaspoon of ginger:

Mix 2 cups of warm water with 1 cup of Quaker Oats (regular kind), 1 tablespoon of butter, 1½ teaspoons of salt, and ⅓ cup of molasses.

Add the yeast mixture to the oats.

Stir in 2 cups of whole-wheat flour and stir 100 strong strokes to blend.

Add:

½   cup of soy flour

½   cup of white flour

¼   cup of wheat germ

Stir well after each addition.

Add an additional 1¼ cups of whole-wheat flour.

Stir well for 3 minutes so that all ingredients are completely blended. This will yield a soft, sticky batter, which is not to be kneaded.

Cover with a warm, wet cloth and place in a warm, draft-free place until the batter has doubled in size—about 1 to 1¼ hours.

Stir down and spoon into three 7¼- by 3½-inch greased bread pans for small loaves, or into two 9- by 5-inch bread pans for larger loaves.

Cover with a wet cloth and allow to double in bulk (around 45 minutes).

When spooning the batter in, it helps to use a wet spoon to fill the pans and push the batter into the corners. The top will look like a plowed field, but this is not important to the taste.

Preheat oven to 350 degrees and bake for 55 minutes.

For a crusty bottom you may place the loaf on the rack of the oven for 5 minutes without the pan (optional).

Cool on a wire rack with a cloth over the bread before serving.

Store in a plastic bag in the refrigerator or for longer periods in the freezer.

CRACKERS

Many crackers contain a great deal of sodium, which will seriously slow your weight loss. Avoid regular saltines and soda crackers.

Check labels, and, if your store does not carry attractive crackers that have a whole grain listed as their first or only ingredient, choose those that list a whole grain, or bran, as a second ingredient. Many brands now offer low-salt choices that are just as tasty as the higher-salt variety, in my opinion. Some of my favorites are Triscuit Hint of Salt, Unsalted Tops Saltines, and RYVITA Dark Rye and Sesame Rye crackers.

CEREALS

With respect to cereals, I hope there is one you like from the following list because they are among the best that you can use in a calorie-restricted diet—they are the high-fiber cereals I refer to in my menus:

40% Bran Flakes	All-Bran Bran	Multi-Bran
Shredded Wheat	Buds	Chex
Original	Puffed Wheat	Corn Bran
Shredded Wheat	Oat Bran	Oatmeal
Bran	Grape-Nuts	
All-Bran Original	Wheat Chex	

The calorie values of these cereals, per serving, will be found on the package. They tend to range between 70 and 110 calories per ounce. Look for cereals that have at least 5 grams of fiber or more per serving.

Milk and Milk Products

Skim milk has virtually no fat and contains about 80 calories per 8 ounces. Low-fat milk will contain about 100 calories for 1 percent butterfat content, and around 120 calories if it has a 2 percent butterfat content. I use low-fat milk because its fat content satisfies hunger for a much longer period of time than does skim milk (and I prefer the flavor). Yogurt is also an excellent choice for dairy and has about the same calorie content as its milk counterparts.

CHEESE

Many herbs, seeds, and spices can be used to advantage with cheese. My favorite herbs are dillweed, rosemary, sage, and thyme. Seeds include caraway, celery, and dill. Certain spices can be sprinkled over cheddar, Monterey Jack, Swiss, or Havarti cheese and then toasted on a slice of whole-wheat bread, in either a regular or a microwave oven. This makes a tasty, toasted, open-faced sandwich for breakfast or lunch. The best spice for cheese toast is chili powder, cumin, or curry powder, plus a dash of cayenne pepper.

Be sure to control your serving size of cheese. Many varieties are high in sodium. Cheddar has about 200 milligrams per ounce, while blue has almost 400 milligrams per ounce. Monterey Jack, Muenster, Tilsit, and Swiss are among the lowest, at around 100 milligrams per ounce.

Try the following Mexican Cheese Toast when the diet calls for 1 slice (about 1 ounce) of cheese and 1 slice of whole-wheat bread.

MEXICAN CHEESE TOAST

1 ounce of cheese (cheddar, Monterey Jack, Swiss)	1 slice of whole-wheat bread
Chili powder	Dash of cayenne (optional)

Slice the cheese thinly so that it covers the bread. Sprinkle generously with chili powder and add a dash of cayenne if you like it hot. This takes less than a minute to melt in a microwave, or you can do it under a broiler, in which case it will take a little longer and bear watching.

Anytime the menu calls for a slice of cheese and a slice of bread, you can combine them to make some form of cheese toast. Vary the recipe by using the other herbs and spices.

The average slice of bread is about 70 calories, while a slice of cheese (about 1 ounce in weight) will generally contain 100 calories. Thus, cheese toast will have approximately 170 calories.

COTTAGE CHEESE PLUS

The Rotation Diet recommends cottage cheese as one of the dairy staples in its menus. Cottage cheese is a very good source of protein, carbohydrate, and calcium. I like cottage cheese with just about any fruit except citrus. If you don't care much for cottage cheese in its plain form, or soon get bored with it, try flavoring it with one or more of the herbs and spices I mentioned under "Cheese" to make Cottage Cheese Plus. Also, in addition to or instead of celery seed, I especially like to sprinkle my cottage cheese with either onion or garlic powder. If you can't get excited about cottage cheese, try Breakstone's Lowfat Cottage Cheese. Participants in the WMP rated Breakstone's a winner in all comparison tests.

Serving size is ½ cup, at about 90 calories per serving.

EGGS

CURRIED UNSTUFFED HARD-BOILED EGG

You can more than double the calories in deviled or stuffed eggs when you add those gobs of mayonnaise. It's unnecessary. Just sprinkle slices of hard-boiled egg with one or more of the following: curry or chili powder, cumin, onion powder, celery seeds, freshly ground black pepper. I find that any of these seasonings will satisfy my palate without adding mayonnaise or salt.

Serving size is 1 egg, at about 80 calories per egg.

Sandwiches

COMBINATION SANDWICH

The label "Combination Sandwich" refers to any combination of ingredients between 2 slices of bread, such as ham (or any slice of meat) and cheese, or spreads with vegetables or cheese.

The way to prepare sandwiches with limited calories is to use lean cuts of meat or fowl, and only limited amounts of dressing. Two slices of bread, with 1 ounce each of meat and cheese, will contain about 295 calories. Mayonnaise is about 33 calories a teaspoon, ketchup is 16 calories a tablespoon, and mustard is negligible. Add *free vegetables* and you have a satisfying lunch for about 350 calories. (Compare the calorie content of this lunch with the 650 or so calories you obtain in the typical fast-food hamburger sandwich. The fast-food hamburger can have as much as five times the fat content of your lean slice of meat, and three to six times more mayonnaise or salad dressing will be used to enhance the flavor.)

For variety, try one of the following spreads. They make especially attractive open-faced sandwiches. Serve with sprouts, or a slice of tomato or cheese, and broil in the oven for a hot sandwich.

Meat Spread

½ pound of cooked meat   2 tablespoons of soy
   or fowl   flour
1 small onion, diced   Herb Salt (p. 147)
¼ cup of wheat germ (or   Freshly ground black
   cooked red beans)   pepper

Blend all ingredients in a food processor. Moisten as needed with ketchup or salad dressing.

Makes about 1¼ cups; serving size is about 2 ounces, or ¼ cup, at about 95 calories per serving.

Crabmeat Spread

1 cup of crabmeat   ½ green pepper, diced
½ cup of celery, diced   1 cup of sprouts
1 small onion, diced   1 cup of low-fat cottage
   Herb Salt (p. 147)   cheese

Mix all ingredients together with enough salad dressing to moisten.

Makes about 3 cups; serving size is about 2 ounces, or ¼ cup, at about 35 calories per serving.

Mexican Bean Spread

This is one of my favorites. It can substitute for a Mexican bean dip, and it is great broiled in the oven covered with a slice of cheese, or tomato, and sprinkled with oregano.

1	can of dark-red kidney beans	⅛	teaspoon of cayenne pepper
1	small onion		Herb Salt (p. 147)
3	tablespoons of ketchup		Freshly ground black pepper

Blend in a food processor, adding more ketchup if needed for desired consistency.

Makes about 1½ cups; serving size is about 2 ounces, or ¼ cup, at about 90 calories per serving.

TUNA- OR SALMON-SALAD SANDWICH

See the recipe for tuna or salmon salad on page 116. With 2 slices of bread, lettuce, and/or sprouts, plus ¼ of the salad recipe, a typical sandwich will contain between 260 and 325 calories, depending on the amount of mayonnaise used.

Soups

SOUP BASE

This is the basic stock that I use for making soup of various kinds, as well as for making rice and boiled potatoes. It is excellent for soaking and cooking beans. By adding only a minimal amount of salt, you can keep the sodium content of your own stock at a fraction of what is contained in commercial soups and bouillons.

Save all chicken and turkey giblets (necks, hearts, gizzards, but *not* livers) and freeze immediately, first trimming skin and any fat from the necks. Hold in your freezer until you have accumulated the parts of 4 to 6 birds. Then:

Place giblets in a deep soup kettle, with enough water to cover (about 8 to 10 cups). Bring to a boil and skim as necessary. When finally clear of scum, add:

1 large bay leaf	Salt and pepper to taste
1 teaspoon each of rosemary, sage, thyme, and tarragon	1 large onion, coarsely chopped
2 large stalks of celery, in 2-inch pieces (include leaves)	2 large carrots, in 2-inch pieces

Throw in any other greens or wilted vegetables you have hanging out in your refrigerator (except for cabbage, broccoli, or cauliflower).

Bring to boil once again, then reduce heat and simmer for at least 2 hours.

Separate giblets and vegetables from water. Blend vegetables and return to stock. Save giblets for low-calorie snacks.

Freeze the stock in 2- to 4-cup plastic containers and use as needed.

THURSDAY'S VEGETABLE SOUP

This soup bears the name it does because I made it for the first time on a Thursday, a day before I was about to do a television show on low-calorie cooking, when the temperature was near zero outdoors. What could be better than a hot cup of soup on such a day?

To 1 cup of soup stock (or commercial low-salt bouillon), throw in a quartered onion, sliced carrot, and a sliced stalk of celery, plus anything else in the way of vegetables that you have left over in the refrigerator (red cabbage will give it a delightful red tint).

Add seasonings to taste—for example, thyme, a few sprigs of rosemary, a touch of parsley, etc.

Each serving of 1 cup contains about 15 to 20 calories; depending on how many vegetables you throw in, you can end up with 2 or 3 cups, at about 40 or 60 calories for the total.

This soup is another food that you can use almost as freely as a *free vegetable* (some of the vegetables that you use may be more than 10 calories a serving).

You can make the soup a little heartier by using some potatoes, and I strongly suggest that you do occasionally. This will make the soup even more filling and satisfy your hunger for longer periods. A small (3½-ounce) potato will add only 90 calories to the entire recipe.

Salads

CREATIVE FRUIT SALAD

This is called Creative Fruit Salad because you use whatever fruits you have on hand, cut them up into chunks, sprinkle with lemon juice to keep the fruit looking fresh and to add a bit of tang, and then add 1 tablespoon of ONE of any of the following:

grated coconut

chopped unsalted nuts (of
  any kind)

raisins or chopped dates

Add a sprinkle of any of the following spices:

cinnamon

nutmeg

allspice

ginger

anise

cardamom

A main-course serving is 2 cups of any combination of fresh fruits plus 1 tablespoon of nuts or raisins. Average calories: about 200 per serving.

CREATIVE CHEF SALAD

	Several large leaves of romaine		Plus choice of additional vegetables
¼	head of any lettuce, shredded	1	egg, quartered (optional)
¼	cup of red cabbage, shredded	1	tomato, quartered
¼	cup of shaved carrots	1	slice of green pepper
1	ounce of Swiss cheese, cut in narrow strips		Lo-Cal Salad Dressing (p. 119)
1	ounce of white-meat turkey or chicken, in strips		Herb Salt (p. 147)
			Freshly ground black pepper

Arrange your selections attractively on the romaine and use 1 to 2 tablespoons of dressing.

The calorie content of this salad will range from 300 to 400, depending on whether you include the egg, and the amount of dressing you use.

DINNER SALAD

For each portion, use:

½	carrot, thinly sliced	¼	cup of shredded red cabbage or
1	stalk of celery, thinly sliced or	4	sliced mushrooms
¼	green pepper, diced lettuce or greens	2	thin slices of sweet red onion

A dinner-size salad bowl of this mixture will contain about 40 calories. Use with No- or Lo-Cal Salad Dressing (p. 119) and flavor with Herb Salt (p. 147) if you like.

TUNA OR SALMON SALAD

1	6½-ounce can of water-packed tuna or salmon	1	large carrot
		2	stalks of celery

Blend in a food processor or blender, adding enough salad dressing or mayonnaise for desired consistency. If you prefer to do the blending by hand, the carrot and celery should be sliced thin, or chopped. Serve with lettuce and tomato, or with 2 slices of bread and sprouts as a sandwich.

Blended with 1 tablespoon of mayonnaise, this makes 3 tuna-salad portions at 136 calories each. If you leave out the mayonnaise, the calories per serving are 103. For salmon-salad portions of the same size, add 30 calories.

SALMON WITH HERBS

Even canned salmon can be interesting when it's dressed in its most complementary herbs. My favorites are thyme, marjoram, and sage—just a dash or two of each. Celery seed goes well too, and so does the mustard vinaigrette dressing I suggest below for the sardines (a bit of mustard and a drop of lemon juice or vinegar). Serve with toast, whole-wheat crackers, and/or a leaf of romaine.

Serving size is 3 ounces, at 156 calories per serving.

SARDINES VINAIGRETTE

I include sardines because they are an excellent low-calorie source of protein and calcium, even when packed in oil. Their nutritional value makes them an excellent addition to the 600/900-calorie rotations. Just drain, and top with a bit of Dijon mustard and a drop of lemon juice or vinegar. Serve on a leaf or two of romaine, and garnish with any of your *free vegetables*.

Serving size is 2 ounces, or about 3 medium-sized sardines, at 88 calories per serving.

SPINACH SALAD

For each serving:

2	cups of fresh spinach, trimmed	1	Bermuda onion, sliced (optional)
3	large mushrooms, sliced	3	slices of green pepper
½	hard-boiled egg, chopped		Lo-cal dressing of your choice (or see p. 119)

Arrange spinach on a large platter, and then layer the other vegetables over it in an attractive manner—a spinach salad is one of the most pleasant salads to behold, especially if you choose to add a few slices of Bermuda onion.

Contains about 115 calories per serving, including the egg. Add 33 calories per tablespoon of Lo-Cal Salad Dressing (p. 119), or check the bottle of any lo-cal dressing of your own. If you wish to keep the calories down, use No-Cal Salad Dressing (p. 119).

LUNCHEON TUNA VINAIGRETTE

I prefer my tuna plain with a few drops of fresh lemon juice or wine vinegar. For extra zest, try canned, water-packed tuna with tarragon vinegar (you can buy this commercially) or use my recipe for No-Cal Salad Dressing, with the addition of tarragon.

Serving size is 3 ounces at 120 calories per serving.

Salad Dressings

COTTAGE-CHEESE DRESSING

½ cup of low-fat cottage cheese

½ cup of plain low-fat yogurt

½ green pepper, chopped

4 radishes, sliced

2 tablespoons of chives

1 tablespoon of poppy seeds

Herb Salt (p. 147) to taste

Mix in a blender or food processor. It is excellent with salads and baked potatoes. For variety, add onions or 2 ounces of blue cheese. (Blue cheese will add about 40 milligrams of sodium to each tablespoonful of this dressing.)

About 12 calories per tablespoon, or 22 calories per tablespoon when blue cheese is added.

NO-CAL SALAD DRESSING

½ cup of wine vinegar

½ teaspoon of Herb Salt (p. 147)

1 tablespoon of fresh chopped parsley

1 clove of garlic, crushed, or ¼ teaspoon of garlic powder

Mix well. Use other herbs and vinegars for variety. Tarragon is one of the best herbs for salad dressings. And, if available, try the fruit vinegars (they are excellent) such as raspberry or strawberry. You may add ¼ to ½ cup of water to this dressing if it is too vinegary for your taste.

LO-CAL SALAD DRESSING

¼ cup of fine olive oil

¼ cup of water

¼ cup of wine or fruit vinegar

1 clove of garlic, crushed

½ teaspoon of salt

1 teaspoon of dried tarragon

Blend by shaking in a jar and letting stand for several hours before its first use. Always shake before using.

Use different herbs for variety.

For extra tang, add 1 teaspoon of Dijon mustard.

About 33 calories per tablespoon. (Don't be concerned about the water in this recipe—it helps spread the flavors and saves calories. Many commercial recipes use water to save calories, just as this one does.)

BALSAMIC NO-CAL DRESSING

¾	cup of water	1½	teaspoons of dried basil
¼	cup of balsamic vinegar	1	tablespoon of fresh parsley, chopped (optional)
3	teaspoons of capers		
2	teaspoons of prepared Dijon mustard		

Put in blender and place on high speed. (Adjust vinegar to taste.)

About 2 calories per tablespoon.

Meats: Beef and Pork

You probably have some favorite ways of preparing meat, and you should feel free to use them if the recipes call for lean cuts and no added fat or oil.

Here are three quick ways of flavoring steak or lean beef patties. Similar seasonings can be used with other cuts of beef.

STEAK AND HAMBURGER TERIYAKI STYLE

Sprinkle a 4-ounce (raw weight) lean beef patty with ground ginger, freshly ground black pepper, just a touch of garlic powder and onion powder, and a teaspoon of soy sauce. Try a low-salt variety of soy sauce if you wish to be more moderate in your salt intake. Pan-broil or oven-broil without added fat. (A 4-ounce patty reduces to 3 ounces during cooking.)

Use the same seasonings with steak, calculating your portion size as directed three paragraphs below.

Variation 1. Italian Seasonings. Sprinkle liberally with garlic powder and onion powder, and your choice of herbs such as oregano, basil, thyme, marjoram, and parsley. Add a touch of freshly ground black pepper. This recipe doesn't need salt, so don't add any until you serve the hamburger and taste it. After turning in the pan, spread hamburger with a teaspoon of ketchup or chili sauce.

Variation 2. Chili Seasonings. Sprinkle liberally with Mexican chili powder, paprika, and a dash of cayenne pepper. Cumin and basil will make interesting additions to the flavor as well. Add salt after tasting at the table.

Lean beef and extra-lean hamburger will average about 55 calories per cooked ounce. Serving size is 3 ounces cooked (165 calories) on the 600/900-calorie rotations, 4½ ounces cooked (248 calories) on the 1200-calorie rotation, and 6 ounces cooked (330 calories) at the higher levels.

STEAK FLAMED IN BRANDY

Flavor your steak with your favorite seasonings and pan-broil. Just before serving, pour 1 ounce of brandy over the steak and light fumes with a match. Let it burn out before serving.

Just about all of the calories in the brandy burn off, so figure about 55 calories an ounce for lean meat.

MARINATED FLANK STEAK

You can use either of the following two marinades with any cut of steak, but I like to use flank steak because it is one of the leanest cuts of meat and the marinade tenderizes it. In addition, the use of either marinade is excellent for outdoor grilling. If you use any other cut of steak, be sure to trim all the visible fat (most of the calories in any cut of steak come from fat, *not* protein).

2	pounds of flank steak	1	bay leaf
1	tablespoon of salad oil	2	cloves of garlic, minced
½	cup of dry white wine	2	teaspoons of chopped chives
1	small onion, minced		
¼	teaspoon of thyme leaves		

Steak must be marinated overnight to obtain the full tenderizing and flavoring effect. Use a covered bowl or two plastic bags (one might leak). (An extra tenderizing and even more flavorful effect can be obtained if you take the trouble to pierce the steak with the tines of a fork on both sides, before putting it in the marinade, at intervals of about a ¼ inch.)

Broil about 4 minutes on each side, basting with marinade as you turn the meat. Use all of the marinade. Slice thinly on the diagonal to serve (it's both attractive and easy for the diner to deal with diagonal cuts); and cover with sauce from the pan. Add salt and pepper to taste at the table.

Here is an Asian marinade that will have you salivating every time you think about it after you have sampled it:

1   tablespoon of salad oil

¼   cup of tamari

¼   cup of dry red wine

4   cloves of garlic, minced

4   scallions, minced

6   whole peppercorns

¼   teaspoon of ground coriander

1-inch cube of fresh ginger, peeled and grated or minced (it must be fresh ginger—the powder just won't give you the flavor of the fresh root)

Marinate overnight and cook as above.

Each 4-ounce serving of cooked flank steak will contain about 220 calories.

Each 2 pounds of steak (raw weight) will yield about 6 servings. The exact number of servings depends on the size you desire, and you must remember that there is about 25 percent shrinkage from the raw to the cooked state.

HERBED PORK

4   lean pork chops, 1 to 1½ inches thick

2   tablespoons of tamari

1   teaspoon of cornstarch or flour

1   clove of garlic, minced

½   teaspoon each of rosemary, thyme, tarragon, oregano, sage, and basil

Salt and freshly ground black pepper to taste

Trim all visible fat. Puncture the chops with the tines of a fork at intervals of about ¼ inch. Rub well with the cornstarch or flour.

Place the tamari, herbs, garlic, and pepper in a shallow bowl and marinate the chops for at least 2 hours (preferably overnight). Be sure the chops are coated on both sides with the marinade and turn two or three times. This marinade is an excellent tenderizer. (Add a little more tamari if there is not enough to coat the chops, and leave a bit remaining in the bottom of your marinating bowl.)

Place chops in a skillet with ½ cup of water, cover, and simmer *very gently* for 45 minutes. Do not boil as this will toughen the meat. Remove chops. Pour off and save the liquid. If you have trimmed the meat well, there will be very little fat on top of the liquid. Remove any that remains.

Return chops to the pan and brown on both sides. When done, place on warm platter. Return liquid to skillet and heat, tasting occasionally to determine how much salt to add. You can add more water to taste, or perhaps ¼ cup of dry white wine (the alcohol will evaporate, leaving the flavor). It takes about 2 to 3 minutes to make this sauce.

Pour over the chops and serve (you might want to save a bit of the sauce for a baked potato if that is also on the menu).

Lamb chops can be made with a similar marinade. However, lamb chops should be pan-broiled in a skillet, uncovered, without water, for about 7 to 8 minutes per side. Remove the chops and add either ½ cup of water or a 50/50 mixture of water and dry red wine to the drippings in the skillet and heat to make a sauce.

The lean meat, separated from all visible fat, will contain about 55 calories per ounce, but unless you do a perfect job of trimming, you should figure about 70 calories per ounce, or about 315 calories for a 4½-ounce serving and 420 calories for a 6-ounce serving.

POT ROAST OF BEEF

This particular roast is made with Italian seasonings.

2   pounds of lean roast (top or bottom round, trimmed) or 2 pounds of flank steak

4   cloves of garlic, minced

2   medium onions, sliced

1   green pepper, sliced

4   stalks of celery, cut in 2-inch pieces

6   large carrots, cut in 2-inch pieces

12   new potatoes

1   bay leaf

1   tablespoon of Italian seasonings*

1   28-ounce can of tomatoes

1   15-ounce can of tomato sauce or puree

2   teaspoons of soy sauce

Dash of Worcestershire sauce

Salt and pepper to taste

Optional: ½ cup of hearty red wine

Place meat in a large roasting pan and cover with minced garlic and slices of onions and green pepper. Place other vegetables and potatoes all around the meat.

Mix the soy sauce and Worcestershire sauce in either the tomatoes or the tomato sauce, and then add both to the roast (together with the wine, if you use it). Add all the other seasonings.

Cook in a slow oven (250 degrees) for 4 to 5 hours, or until meat falls apart when prodded with the tines of a fork.

* Use a commercial Italian seasoning, or mix your own from oregano, basil, marjoram, tarragon, and thyme, about ½ teaspoon each, plus ¼ teaspoon of rosemary.

Makes 6 to 8 servings (3 to 4 ounces of meat, cooked), which, with vegetables, will average 275 to 325 calories per serving, respectively.

FOWL

ALMOND CHICKEN

3   pounds of chicken breasts, skinned and boned

⅓   cup of tamari

1-inch cube of fresh ginger, finely minced (or 1 teaspoon of dry ground ginger)

3   cloves of garlic, finely minced (or 1 teaspoon of powder)

½   cup of whole-wheat flour

½   cup of finely ground almonds

½   teaspoon of salt

½   teaspoon of pepper

2   tablespoons of peanut or corn oil

In a large bowl, combine the tamari, ginger, and garlic. Cut the chicken into bite-size chunks and marinate in the tamari mixture while you prepare the other ingredients.

In another bowl, combine flour, almonds, and the rest of the seasonings. Add this to the chicken and toss until the chicken is coated with the flour mixture.

Heat the oil in a wok or large skillet on high heat. When the oil is hot, add the chicken, and turn the heat down to medium. Cook covered, stirring often, about 20 minutes.

This goes well with rice and a green vegetable.

Makes 8 servings at 223 calories per serving, not including the rice and vegetables.

BAKED CHICKEN

There are countless ways to prepare poultry, and I will present several other recipes in addition to the simplest baking recipes later in this book. During the 600/900-calorie rotations of your diet it is probably best to keep the recipes simple, in order to be sure a few hundred extra calories don't sneak into your daily diet. Oven baking is one of those simple but delicious ways to prepare chicken.

Line a baking pan with foil and lay out the pieces of a small fryer. Flavor with your favorite seasonings and bake at 300 degrees for approximately 1 hour. Skin before eating (much of the flavor of the seasonings will have penetrated to the flesh of the chicken during baking; however, add more at the table, if desired).

Try the following different combinations of seasonings for variety.

Variation 1. Sprinkle liberally with onion, garlic powder, and Herb Salt (page 147). Or make your own selection of herbs, using one or more of the following: marjoram, oregano, rosemary, tarragon, or thyme. Add freshly ground black pepper.

Variation 2. Sprinkle liberally with chili powder, paprika, and add a dash of cayenne pepper. Add salt at the table after tasting.

Variation 3. Calories are significantly less if the chicken is skinned *before* baking. But skinning prior to cooking creates a problem since the meat is likely to dry out. You can prevent this by coating the skinned chicken with a basting sauce made from ½ cup of ketchup, 2 tablespoons of tamari, and 2 ounces of sherry. Then sprinkle with other herbs of your choice. (Additional salt is not needed because of the tamari.) Cover the chicken lightly with a piece of aluminum foil for about half of the actual cooking time and it will stay moist.

White meat baked without the skin is about 45 calories an ounce, dark meat is about 50. On 600/900-calorie rotations, the serving size is 3 ounces cooked (135 and 150 calories for white and dark meat, respectively). On the 1200-calorie rotation, the serving size is 4½ ounces (208 and 225 calories for white and dark meat, respectively). On 1500- and 1800-calorie rotations, the serving size is 6 ounces (270 and 300 calories for white and dark meat, respectively). Basting sauce will add between 15 and 30 calories per serving, depending on size.

LEMON-BAKED CHICKEN

About 3½ pounds of chicken pieces, skinned

¼ cup of lemon juice

1 onion, cut into chunks

1 clove of garlic, finely diced

¼ teaspoon of thyme

¼ teaspoon of marjoram

¼ teaspoon of freshly ground black pepper

1 tablespoon of fresh parsley, chopped

Combine all ingredients in a 3-quart casserole dish and marinate for at least an hour, covered in the refrigerator. Stir occasionally.

Bake, covered, in a preheated oven at 350 degrees for 1½ hours.

Serves 4 to 6. See Baked Chicken for the calorie count. (This chicken is so good as a leftover you may wish to double the recipe.)

CHICKEN TOMASI

This dish is adapted from a traditional Hungarian recipe. We are not sure it originated in the town of Tomasi, but we like the name!

3 pounds of chicken pieces, skinned	¼ teaspoon of cayenne
2 teaspoons of butter	½ cup of chicken or vegetable bouillon
1 medium onion, chopped	1 cup of plain yogurt
1 clove of garlic, minced	¼ cup of low-fat milk
5 teaspoons of paprika	Salt and black pepper to taste

Melt 1 teaspoon of butter in a large saucepan and brown the chicken pieces. Remove the chicken from the pan and drain on paper towels on a platter.

Melt the remaining butter in the pan, and sauté the onion and garlic, covering the saucepan, until the onions are clear.

Place the chicken back in the pan, sprinkle with paprika and cayenne, and pour the bouillon in. Simmer, covered, until the chicken is tender.

Again, remove the chicken from the pan, and remove the pan from the burner. Let the bouillon cool for several minutes. Cooling is essential to prevent the dairy products from curdling.

When the bouillon is lukewarm, stir in the yogurt and the milk until smooth. Replace the skillet over low heat, add salt and pepper to taste, and put the chicken back in.

Reheat until hot—but do not let the sauce boil!

The chicken contains approximately 300 calories for a 6-ounce serving. Add 10 calories for each tablespoon of sauce.

Serves 6 to 8.

Fish

POACHED FISH FILLETS

Poaching is about the simplest low-calorie way to prepare fish fillets as well as fish steaks, such as salmon or halibut.

2 pounds of fish fillets or steaks

1 cup of dry white wine

2 cups of water

1 tablespoon of chopped fresh parsley

1 bay leaf

1 lemon, thinly sliced

Herb Salt to taste (p. 147)

Sliced lemon and sprigs of parsley for garnish

Optional ingredients:

1 onion, thinly sliced

1 carrot, thinly sliced

1 cup of bottled clam juice

Combine wine, water, chopped parsley, bay leaf, thinly sliced lemon, and Herb Salt, plus optional ingredients, and bring to a boil in a saucepan. Reduce heat and simmer for 30 minutes. Strain.

Divide fish into portions of approximately 4 to 8 ounces, depending on what your daily menu calls for (the weight will be reduced by 25 percent during baking). Place in a casserole dish with the wine-water mixture. Cover and bake at 300 degrees for about 20 minutes, or until fish flakes when tested with a fork.

Remove fish to a warm platter with a couple of tablespoons of its broth and cover with foil to keep moist. Place the remainder of the broth in the saucepan and heat to reduce by half.

Pour over the fish before serving and garnish with additional lemon slices and parsley.

Shortcut Method: I have had excellent luck with this dish using a shortcut method that takes only about 5 minutes of preparation once you gather the ingredients.

Place your fish in the center of a piece of aluminum foil large enough to fold over the fish. Place the foil and fish in a baking pan. Season with Herb Salt and any of the other ingredients from the above recipe that you like. Cut the liquid ingredients in the above recipe to ½ cup of white wine, ½ cup of water, and (optional) ½ cup of clam juice. Pour directly over the fish and fold the foil tightly to make a perfect seal.

Place in a preheated 300-degree oven and bake for about 30 minutes, or until fish flakes when tested with a fork.

Let the fish cool a bit before serving. Taste the bouillon and reduce, if necessary, to obtain the strength of flavor you prefer. Then pour over the fish before serving.

Fish fillets will average about 50 calories an ounce, cooked. Serving size is 3 ounces cooked on 600/900-calorie rotations, 4½ ounces cooked on 1200 calories, and 6 ounces cooked on higher intakes.

Serves 6 to 8 (depending on where you are in the Rotation Diet).

BAKED FISH FILLETS

1½ pounds of fillets (sole, flounder, etc.)	2 tablespoons of fresh parsley, chopped
1 tablespoon of oil	1 lemon (6 wedges)
1 tablespoon of lemon juice	Salt and freshly ground black pepper to taste

In the bottom of a shallow baking or broiling pan, spread the oil, lemon juice, and pepper. Swish the fish around in the pan, coating both sides. Sprinkle with parsley.

Broil 3 to 4 minutes on each side or until the edges are browned. Serve with lemon wedges, and add salt to taste at the table.

See Poached Fish Fillets for the calorie counts.

Serves 4 to 6 (depending on where you are in the Rotation Diet).

BAKED OR BROILED RAINBOW TROUT

4 small trout (about ¾ pound each)	Freshly ground black pepper to taste
1 tablespoon of oil	
Herb Salt to taste (p. 147)	

Preheat oven to 500 degrees. Pour oil into aluminum-lined baking pan, swish fish around well in the oil, season, and bake for about 12 minutes, or until fish flakes easily with a fork. You may broil if you prefer.

If you like your fish with garlic and onion flavorings, sprinkle with garlic powder and onion powder before baking.

Serves 4. Edible portion, approximately 4 ounces, will contain about 125 calories.

ROYAL INDIAN SALMON

- 4 salmon steaks, 1 inch thick
- ¼ cup of chicken or vegetable bouillon
- 2 tablespoons of lemon juice
- ½ teaspoon of fennel seeds, crushed
- ¼ teaspoon of cumin
- ¼ teaspoon of ground coriander
- Dash of salt
- Freshly ground black pepper

Place the steaks in a shallow glass pan. Pour the bouillon and the lemon juice over the steaks. Add the seasonings.

Marinate, covered, in the refrigerator for at least 2 hours, turning the steaks occasionally.

To cook, place the steaks on a foil-covered broiling pan. Spoon 2 teaspoons of the marinade on top of each steak. Place under the broiler for 6 to 8 minutes, or until slightly brown on the edges. Turn steaks over, spoon on the remaining marinade, and broil for an additional 6 to 8 minutes.

A 6-ounce serving will contain approximately 330 calories.

Note: This dish has a delicate, aristocratic flavor—not too spicy or hot in the way many people expect Indian cooking to be.

Vegetarian

EGGPLANT CASSEROLE

This hearty dish uses my favorite vegetarian burger, Morning-star Farms, which I find in the freezer section of my grocery. These vegetarian burgers have a good consistency and flavor, and I don't miss the meat that was called for in the original recipe.

1	onion, chopped		Black pepper to taste
4	cloves of garlic, chopped	¼	teaspoon of salt
			Oregano to taste
1	bell pepper, chopped	1	can (15 ounces) of tomato sauce
1	tablespoon of olive oil		
1	package of MorningStar Farms Grillers Original veggie burgers	1	large eggplant, cut into ½-inch slices
		1½	cups of grated cheddar cheese
1	tablespoon of flour		

In a medium saucepan, sauté the onion, garlic, and bell pepper in oil on medium-low heat. Meanwhile, microwave the veggie burgers, following directions on the package, then chop them. When the onion is translucent, add the veggie burgers, flour, spices, and tomato sauce to the saucepan, and heat through. In a greased 2-quart casserole, layer half the eggplant slices. Top with half of the veggie mixture, then half of the cheese. Repeat layers. Bake at 350 degrees for 35 to 45 minutes, until bubbly. Remove from oven and let stand for about 5 minutes before serving.

Makes 8 servings at 200 calories per serving.

Pasta

MY FAVORITE PASTA

Garlic and Clam Sauce

This is a favorite at our house.

This is an unusual but very tasty garlic and clam sauce that combines additional vegetables with the clams so that a large serving can use a bit less spaghetti or linguini, and a little more sauce, with fewer calories per portion. *I use Rice noodles*

2	tablespoons of fine olive oil		Dash of cayenne
4	cloves of garlic, minced	2	6- or 7-ounce cans of minced clams
½	cup of chopped onion	½	cup of chopped green peppers
½	pound of mushrooms, sliced		Salt and freshly ground black pepper to taste
1½	teaspoons of dried thyme leaves		
2	tablespoons of chopped fresh parsley		

Sauté the onion, green peppers, and garlic in the olive oil until translucent (add a little water and cover if necessary during this process). Add the mushrooms and continue heating in the covered saucepan for about 3 minutes. Add the remaining ingredients, including all the liquid that comes with the clams, and heat until hot in the covered saucepan.

Makes 4 servings (approximately 70 calories each).

Serve with 1 cup of spaghetti or linguini (2 ounces dry; about 200 calories) and Parmesan cheese (optional).

Total calories per serving are 270. Add 50 calories per table-spoon of Parmesan cheese.

Meat Sauce

1 pound of extra-lean chopped meat	1 stalk of celery, chopped
1 large onion, chopped	1 green pepper, chopped
1 28-ounce can of tomatoes	1 teaspoon of chili powder
1 6-ounce can of tomato paste	½ teaspoon of oregano
1 tablespoon of Worcestershire sauce	½ teaspoon of basil
	Salt and pepper to taste

Brown the first four ingredients (if you have bought extra-lean beef, there will be no fat to pour off). Add the remaining ingredients and bring to a boil. Reduce heat immediately and simmer, uncovered, for about an hour or until sauce reaches desired consistency. You may add a small amount of water to taste, or ¼ cup of dry red wine, during cooking.

Makes 6 servings of about 125 calories each.

Total calories are about 325 when served with 1 cup of cooked spaghetti. Add 50 calories per tablespoon of Parmesan cheese, if used.

Vegetables

The best ways to prepare most vegetables to keep the calorie content at a minimum are steamed, boiled in a very small amount of water, and cooked in a microwave, according to its directions. During the 600/900-calorie rotations, we use no fats or other additions that will increase the calories unnecessarily—we concentrate on herbs. At higher intake levels you can dress your vegetables up with small amounts of fat and other caloric additions.

All vegetables can be eaten plain, or with just a sprinkle of salt (or, better, Herb Salt, page 147) and freshly ground black pepper, if you desire. The following recipes add a bit of interest—you may not have considered how herbs and spices can turn the ordinary into the exotic. When you use herbs and spices for seasoning, you will find it easy to reduce or eliminate both salt and fat in your cooking.

Remember that most vegetables are at their nutritious best when eaten raw. While I include tasty ways of cooking the vegetables in the Rotation Diet, you will do well to eat one vegetable raw each day. And cooked vegetables are best when served crisp.

ACORN SQUASH

For baking, cut in half lengthwise, spoon out seeds, and bake face down on aluminum foil at 350 degrees for about 45 minutes, or until tender. Season with salt and pepper to taste at the table. Try a sprinkle of cloves, ginger, or nutmeg for variety.

Serves 2 at 56 calories per half of squash.

ASPARAGUS

Caraway Asparagus

If you use fresh asparagus, cut off the tough part of the stalk and cook the spears in a small amount of water for about 12 minutes or until tender. You can also steam asparagus if you prefer, or use your microwave according to directions. The texture of the tips is best preserved by steaming the asparagus standing upright and covered in a deep saucepan. Peel back an inch or so of the outer stalks before placing them in the saucepan. Add about ½ teaspoon of caraway seeds for each cup of asparagus, plus freshly ground black pepper to taste. (Follow directions on the package for frozen asparagus.)

Cold Dijon Asparagus

Mix 1 tablespoon of Dijon mustard with 1 tablespoon of plain yogurt and ¼ teaspoon of tarragon. Spread over chilled asparagus. Add salt and freshly ground black pepper to taste.

Serving size is 1 cup at 18 calories. Add 8 calories for the Dijon dressing.

GREEN BEANS ALMONDINE

1 10-ounce package of frozen green beans	2 tablespoons of slivered almonds
¼ cup of water	
Dash of salt and pepper	

Cook green beans in water until crispy tender, add remaining ingredients, and simmer for an additional 5 minutes.

Makes 4 servings of ½ cup at 38 calories per serving.

GREEN BEANS WITH CHIVES

1 pound of fresh green beans (2 10-ounce packages frozen)	1 tablespoon of chopped chives (or scallions)
2 tablespoons of chopped fresh parsley	½ tablespoon of Herb Salt (p. 147)

Steam or simmer (in ¼ cup of water) unseasoned beans until tender (or follow directions for your microwave). Sprinkle with other ingredients just before serving.

Variations. Beans can be made with ½ pound of mushrooms, 1 large sliced onion, or 1 can of baby onions, without changing the calorie value of a ½-cup serving to any great extent.

Makes 8 servings of ½ cup at 18 calories per serving.

GINGERED BEETS

You can use canned baby beets, or cook the beets yourself, leaving on about 1 inch of the stem and root ends. Small beets will take about ½ hour to cook in boiling water, or cook them in your microwave according to the manufacturer's instructions for cooking vegetables.

Drain most of the liquid from the beets, and sprinkle lightly with ground ginger (about ¼ teaspoon per ½ cup) before serving.

You can add a couple of tablespoons of cider vinegar if you want some extra zing. Top with a tablespoon of chopped fresh parsley.

Serving size is ½ cup at 29 calories per serving.

BROCCOLI

Broccoli is one of my favorite vegetables. It not only tastes good, but it's a powerhouse when it comes to nutritional value—plenty of vitamins A and C, plus fiber. Broccoli is also a good source of calcium and iron. It should become one of your vegetable staples.

Broccoli is excellent when cooked in the microwave, steamed, or simmered in ¼ cup of water or bouillon until it can be penetrated with the tines of a fork but is still crisp. If you don't care much for broccoli without a sauce, just sprinkle each serving with a teaspoon of Parmesan cheese and you have the 600/900-calorie rotation version of Broccoli au Gratin.

Serving size is ½ cup at 30 calories per serving; add about 15 calories for the cheese.

BROCCOLI WITH BLACK OLIVES

1	large bunch of broccoli (about 1½ pounds)	4	tablespoons of Parmesan cheese
1	tablespoon of olive oil		Salt and pepper to taste
1	clove of garlic, minced		
2	ounces of pitted black olives		

Cook broccoli in a small amount of water for 10 minutes (or in a microwave according to directions). Drain. Sauté garlic in olive oil until lightly brown. Add broccoli and cook over low heat for 5 minutes (do not overcook). Add olives and heat 2 more minutes. Serve immediately and sprinkle with cheese. Add salt and pepper at the table.

Serves 4 at 90 calories per serving.

CARROTS

In my own diet, carrots run a close second to broccoli as my favorite vegetable. I like carrots sliced and cooked in the microwave with nothing but a bit of water (follow your own microwave recipe). Dill and chives make good seasonings.

Carrots a l'Orange

For this variation, add 1 tablespoon of slivered orange peel to each cup of slivered or sliced carrots before cooking. Add Herb Salt (page 147) to taste after serving.

And, of course, in place of the orange, you can use 1 tablespoon of fresh (1 teaspoon of dried) dillweed or 2 tablespoons of chives or chopped scallions for variety.

Serving size is ½ cup at 23 calories per serving.

CARROTS WITH ONIONS

3 cups of carrots, sliced	Salt, pepper, and fresh parsley to taste
1 onion, chopped	
¼ cup of water	

Place ingredients in saucepan, bring to a boil, and then simmer gently until cooked.

Makes 6 servings at 27 calories per serving.

BRAISED CARROTS AND CELERY

The word *braise* refers to a method of cooking in fat, with very little moisture. Naturally, when it comes to weight management, the worst thing you can do in preparing meals is to use even a drop more fat than you need for flavoring. My "braising" is done in the microwave, or in a small amount of water on top of the stove.

4 carrots, cut in ¼-inch slices

4 stalks of celery, cut in 2-inch slices

1 teaspoon of fresh chives (optional)

¼ cup of water

2 teaspoons of olive oil or butter

Place carrots, celery, and chives (if desired) in saucepan with water. Bring to a boil, reduce heat, and let simmer until just tender. Pour off water and mix in oil or butter. When using a microwave, follow the directions that come with your oven.

Makes 4 servings at about 25 calories per serving.

SAVORY STEAMED CAULIFLOWERETS

Cut a medium-size head of cauliflower into 2-inch flowerets, and, for each cup of cauliflower, sprinkle with ½ teaspoon of oregano and ½ teaspoon of savory. Steam until tender.

Serving size is 1 cup at 30 calories per serving.

OLD THYMEY PEAS

Maybe you remember the old folk song Simon and Garfunkel made famous in the sixties: "Scarborough Fair." Here's a recipe that uses all the lovely herbs mentioned in that song.

1 package (10½ ounces) of frozen peas, or 1½ cups fresh	½ teaspoon of sage
	½ teaspoon of rosemary
1 teaspoon of parsley	½ teaspoon of thyme

Cook peas in ¼ cup of water until barely tender. Add seasonings and cook 1 minute more before serving.

Variation. Peas go well with a squeeze of lemon and a pinch of basil (about ⅙ of a lemon and ½ teaspoon of basil per ½ cup). Add salt and pepper to taste.

Serving size for either recipe is ½ cup at 57 calories per serving.

PEAS AND BABY ONIONS

1 package (10½ ounces) of frozen peas, or 1½ cups fresh	1 tablespoon of butter
	Herb Salt (p. 147)
1 small can of baby onions, or 1 large onion, sliced	Freshly ground black pepper to taste

Fresh onions should be sautéed in butter until translucent. Add peas and ¼ cup of water. Cook until tender.

If using canned onions, cook peas first until tender; add onions and butter, and warm.

This is a traditional dish with baked or poached fish. It is especially complementary to salmon.

Makes 4 servings of ½ cup at 75 calories per serving.

BROWN OR WILD RICE

1   cup of brown or wild rice

½   tablespoon of butter or oil

2   cups of bouillon (meat or vegetable)

Other seasonings to taste— for example, 1 tablespoon of chopped chives, scallions, or Herb Salt (p. 147), depending on the bouillon

Melt butter in saucepan, add rice, and stir until rice is coated. Add bouillon, cover, and bring to boil. Reduce heat and simmer gently for 45 minutes, or until all of the liquid has been absorbed.

The rice will expand to 2 cups in volume and provide four ½-cup servings, which, prepared in this way, will contain about 105 calories each.

SPINACH AND BROCCOLI CASSEROLE

2   10-ounce packages of frozen spinach (chopped)

1   10-ounce package of frozen broccoli (chopped)

½   cup of water

1   can of mushroom soup

½   cup of seasoned bread crumbs

½	cup of grated Parmesan cheese	1	teaspoon each of garlic and onion powder
½	cup of grated cheddar cheese	½	cup of low-fat milk
			Salt and pepper to taste

Cook broccoli and spinach in water until completely thawed (but not cooked). Stir in remaining ingredients, place in large casserole dish, and cover with seasoned bread crumbs. Bake at 350 degrees for 35 to 40 minutes.

Makes about 12 servings of ½ cup at approximately 85 calories per serving.

This is an excellent dish as a main course. Just double or triple the serving size, and calculate the calories appropriately.

STIR-FRY SPINACH (OR OTHER GREENS)

1	pound of fresh spinach (or other greens)	Herb Salt to taste (p. 147)
1	tablespoon of oil (olive oil preferred)	Freshly ground black pepper to taste
1	medium onion, sliced thin	

Wash and drain greens. Heat oil in skillet and sauté onions for 1 minute. Add greens and stir until leaves are wilted and greens are hot—about 1 minute more on medium heat.

Serve with a squeeze of lemon or a sprinkle of grated cheese.

Makes 4 servings at about 60 calories per serving.

BAKED TOMATO

2	fresh tomatoes	1	tablespoon of Parmesan cheese
1	clove of garlic, minced		
¼	teaspoon of tarragon		Freshly ground black pepper to taste
¼	teaspoon of basil		

Slice tomatoes in half. Place in shallow baking pan, flat side up. Combine seasonings and cheese, and sprinkle over tomatoes. Bake at 350 degrees for about 30 minutes, or until tender.

Makes 4 servings at about 28 calories per serving.

STIR-FRY VEGETABLES

If you are already experienced in stir-frying, do your vegetables in the way you like them (as long as you keep the fat content down).

The following method of skillet frying comes close to duplicating the results obtained with a wok.

1	thinly sliced green pepper	½	cup of chopped cabbage
4	large carrots (½-inch pieces)	1	pound of fresh greens
2	medium onions, thinly sliced		Pinch of marjoram and thyme
3	cloves of garlic, chopped	2	tablespoons of soy sauce
4	stalks of celery (2-inch pieces)		Freshly ground black pepper
1	tablespoon of butter or oil	2	tablespoons grated cheddar or other cheese

Melt butter in skillet on low heat as you begin to slice your vegetables. I add to the skillet, as I slice them, green pepper, carrots, onions, garlic, and celery, in that order, stirring occasionally. Increase heat to medium for 2 to 3 minutes, then add cabbage and greens, and marjoram and thyme. Cook on medium to medium-high heat, stirring almost continuously, until greens have wilted but other vegetables are still crisp. Add soy sauce and pepper to taste.

Serve with Brown or Wild Rice (page 144), which you will have started about 1 hour before the stir-fry, and top with grated cheese.

Serves four, with each serving containing about 110 calories. Add about 90 calories for each ½ cup of plain cooked brown rice and 100 calories for the cheese. Add additional calories if rice is cooked with any added fat.

HERB SALT

½   teaspoon of basil
¼   teaspoon of dill
¼   teaspoon of salt
¼   teaspoon of thyme
¼   teaspoon of celery seed
¼   teaspoon of dried parsley

Combine ingredients and grind with a mortar and pestle. Store in a small herb jar. Experiment with your own combination of herbs. You will soon find that Herb Salt is an excellent substitute for plain salt, and instead of about 2000 to 2200 milligrams of sodium per teaspoon, it has only 285 milligrams. Thus, a sprinkle of Herb Salt will give you perhaps 30 or 40 milligrams of sodium, rather than about seven times that much (200 to 300 milligrams) if you were to use plain salt.

To make a tasty NO SALT seasoning, use all of the above seasonings except the salt and add ⅛ teaspoon of powdered garlic and ⅛ teaspoon of ground black pepper.

CUSTOMIZING THE ROTATION DIET TO SUIT YOUR PERSONAL TASTES

The daily menus for the Rotation Diet have been developed to provide maximum nutritional value at all calorie levels. By sticking closely to the suggested menus, you are most likely to remain at the planned caloric levels and maximize your weight loss. But you can make substitutions provided you stay within the same food group and keep to the recommended portion sizes, so substitute a vegetable for a vegetable, a fruit for a fruit, and so on.

If you substitute foods during the diet, make sure you use the correct serving sizes whether they are identical (as with vegetables, fruit, and meat, fish, or fowl) or equivalent (with milk products, for example, 1 ounce of hard cheese = ½ cup of low-fat cottage cheese).

You should remember, however, that your nutritional needs are best served by eating a wide variety of foods. For example, vary the color of the vegetables you eat, and include different starches.

There is another potential value to including a wide variety of foods: variety in your choices of foods will ensure that you do not take in large amounts of any given preservative or particular pesticides used in growing a specific food product. You also won't get tired of eating the same foods over and over again.

You don't need to be overly picky about which substitutions are most closely equivalent in calories. It's just not worth your effort to be concerned about 5 or 10 calories, more or less. And as for other nutritional values, you will do best if you choose foods that are similar to each other as substitutions. Consider vegetables of different colors as a group, and substitute one red, orange, or yellow vegetable for another in that group. For example, substitute broccoli for green beans, or arugula for spinach. Just remember the wide-variety principle, and do not continually eat just one or two foods from a given category.

Skipping Meals, Combining Meals, Reversing the Order of Meals

Do you have to follow the menus exactly, or can you eat breakfast for dinner and vice versa? Many people in the WMP juggled the foods around in any given day to please themselves, and it seemed to work out very well. But to be sure that you are obtaining adequate nutrition, make substitutions from the appropriate categories and think in terms of whether, over a week at a time, you have consumed the number of foods in each of the food categories (vegetables, fruits, grains, milk products, protein foods) that you would have consumed had you closely followed the menus. If you wait until evening to eat most of your food for the day, there may be a tendency to overeat, and this will interfere with weight loss.

You will also have little opportunity to burn off calories in activity, since you will soon be going to sleep.

If you have unusual hours, try eating the meals in the order that they would have fit into your workday (breakfast first, etc.), and then make alterations if this doesn't turn out to be satisfactory.

Most alterations in the daily eating patterns will not make a great deal of difference. During the 600-calorie rotation, just have two servings of a grain product, two servings of a milk product, two different vegetables, two different fruits, and about 3 ounces of lean meat, fish, or fowl. That's about as simple as I can make it!

During the 900-calorie rotations, add another grain product and another serving of lean meat, fish, or fowl. There is also room for 1 teaspoon of fat or oil for seasoning or spread.

During the 1200-calorie rotation, make it a total of four grain products, two milk products, at least two different fruits and two different vegetables, and two servings of lean meat, fish, or fowl. And you also have room for 1 tablespoon of fat or oil for seasoning or spread.

Vegetarian Substitutions

Vegetarians can use the Rotation Diet by substituting a complementary protein dish composed of combinations of legumes, grains, seeds, and nuts for meat, fish, or fowl. A combination of a grain with a legume will provide the most complete protein with the fewest calories. A soy product such as tofu can also be substituted any time a food of animal origin is called for in the menus. Adding a small amount of cheese to plant foods will increase the quality of the available protein. A ½ cup of beans with a ½ cup of rice will approximate the caloric value of a 3-ounce serving of lean meat (cooked).

DIET DRINKS AND SUGAR DRINKS

I hope there is one thing I can persuade you to do during the Rotation Diet, and that is to give up drinking diet drinks for the entire three weeks. I want you to see whether imbibing diet drinks is keeping alive your taste for sugary foods, and ultimately leading you to overeat sweets that contain calories. I have not yet met a person who is completely satisfied with the use of artificial sweeteners and who doesn't periodically overindulge on "the real thing" in a way that is disastrous for weight control.

Diet drinks may be deadening your sensitivity to sweetness, as it did for many in the WMP. It can lead you to require more than the normal amount of sweetness to satisfy your palate. If you decide to give up the use of artificial sweeteners (except for an occasional stick of gum), in a matter of just a few weeks your tastebuds will be satisfied by the inherent sugar of fruit and vegetables, and it should be easier for you to stick with your diet or to increase your intake of more nutritious foods. Cutting out the use of all artificial sweeteners may turn out to be a crucial factor in your efforts to control your weight.

Forty-eight years ago, I gave up artificial sweeteners, except for that occasional stick of gum. I add no sugar to any beverage other than a teaspoonful to a large glass of ice tea. I use only small amounts of sugar in baking, usually half or less of what is called for in the recipe. I have never found it necessary to make compensatory alterations in the other ingredients. Compared with my taste for sweets when I was a fat man, my sensitivity to sweetness has increased to the point that most sweetened, processed cold cereals, for example, even Grape-Nuts, taste too sweet to me, even without added sugar. Dried fruits such as raisins, dates, prunes, figs, and apricots are at the limit of my tolerance for sweetness. It's now possible for me to enjoy a single bar of candy without turning on an insatiable yearning. The only time I may exceed that is when a friend who frequently travels to Europe comes back and leaves a pound of the most exquisite Belgian chocolate on the doorstep. My wife and I open the box after a festive meal, and I have been known to down 2 or 3 ounces at a single sitting.

How to Use Sugar

While white table sugar (sucrose) is found naturally in many foods, it has only been freely available in its processed form since the late nineteenth century. Considering that the human capacity to deal with foods as they are found in our natural environments has evolved over two million years, I think it is safe to say that our bodies are not designed to deal with unadulterated sugar. You should avoid using sugar or an artificial sweetener except as a minor ingredient in a recipe containing other ingredients.

There is also a problem with undiluted fruit juice such as apple juice. Although fruit juice is more nutritious than soft drinks, there is a great danger that the taste can encourage us to overdo our intake of it as well as other sugary drinks. Too high a quantity of such drinks seems to be associated with an increase in childhood obesity.

The main ingredients in foods that cause us to overeat are fat combined with sugar, or fat combined with salt. Keeping our appetites under control when faced with an abundance of these foods in our environment is the great challenge for overweight people. But there are ways you can learn to do this, and I will discuss them at length in Chapters 9 and 10.

THE NUTRITIONAL VALUE OF THE ROTATION DIET

The Rotation Diet has been designed to approximate the Recommended Dietary Allowances (RDAs) of known major vitamins and minerals over the entire twenty-one-day period of the diet. The same is true of the suggestions I will make for the maintenance diet.

At the level of 1200 calories and above (including my recommendations for the maintenance diet), the proportions of calories from carbohydrate, protein, and fat are within the range suggested in the 2010 Dietary Guidelines for Americans. For adults, the range for carbohydrate is 45 to 65 percent, for protein 10 to 35 percent, and for fat 20 to 35 percent. With the inclusion of *free vegetables* and *safe fruit*s the proportions for the 600/900-calorie days also fall within these ranges.

VITAMIN SUPPLEMENTS

In spite of the nutritional value of the Rotation Diet, it may be important for you to use a multiple vitamin and mineral supplement while you are on it. Substitutions during the diet may change your intake of certain nutrients. For example, if you do not include milk in your diet, and do not like sardines and salmon from a can, but instead substitute cottage cheese or some other cheese as a calcium source, your intake of calcium will be relatively low. Although this is not likely to be dangerous on a temporary basis, it might be in the long run. If you do not take in enough calcium to provide for your daily needs, your body leeches it from your bones, gradually weakening them. Then, when you reach a more advanced age, you may be more susceptible to osteoporosis than you would have been with an adequate intake. Thus, I think it would be wise to include a calcium supplement in the form of calcium gluconate, calcium lactate, calcium citrate, or calcium carbonate. The last form—calcium carbonate—can be obtained easily and cheaply by eating one Tums tablet each day. Each Tums tablet supplies 500 milligrams of calcium, which, together with the other sources of calcium in the daily menus, will easily bring your intake up to the RDA for this nutrient.

In addition, if you don't care for red meat, your intake of some of the B vitamins and iron may be low, since red meat tends to be a major source of these nutrients in most American diets. Other meat products or vegetables may not be as rich in these nutrients, and lack of them could leave you feeling weak and lethargic.

Furthermore, while on a reduced-calorie diet, the body's need for vitamins and minerals may change. Recent research indicates that vigorous exercise may increase one's needs for certain B vitamins and iron, and this may occur as you become more active. A multiple vitamin and mineral tablet will take care of any increased need.

What Brand Is Best?

I recommend that you visit your drugstore and choose the house brand of a multiple vitamin and mineral tablet that contains, in

general, amounts that approximate the RDAs of the major vitamins and minerals. I would not get anything with higher dosages
than the RDAs because too much of certain nutrients may also
be bad for you. The store brand of a vitamin and mineral supplement is likely to cost about five cents per tablet (versus up to
twenty-five cents for specialty brands that are no better in terms
of their nutritional contents). Discuss adding supplements to your
diet with your physician or nutritionist, and get your druggist's
help in choosing the appropriate tablet. And don't be concerned
if a few of the nutrients are not exactly at the 100 percent level of
the RDAs in the information provided on the label. Just be sure
that you avoid megadoses, and ask the druggist to guide you if
you are uncertain.

SHOPPING LIST FOR WOMEN'S MENUS
OF THE ROTATION DIET

Here is a shopping list to make it easy for you to buy exactly what
you will need for the Rotation Diet. I am not entering quantities
for you; enter your own in the space provided in case you want to
buy enough for the family, or for another person who is going on
the Rotation Diet with you. Look at the Week 1 menus, decide on
any substitutions, and add them to this list.

In addition, it is a good idea to check the recipes that are suggested for each day in case you happen to be out of any of the
items you will need for cooking.

WEEK 1 AND WEEK 3

Fruit

Grapefruit   ____

Apples   ____

Bananas   ____

Berries (in season)   ____

Cantaloupe   ____

Other (for *safe fruit*)   ____

     ____

Grains

Whole-wheat bread   ____

Whole-wheat crackers
(low salt)   ____

Breakfast cereal   ____

     ____

     ____

Dairy Products

Milk (skim or low-fat)   ____

     ____

Cottage cheese (low-fat)   ____

Hard cheese   ____

Miscellaneous

Mayonnaise (optional)   ____

     ____

No-cal or lo-cal dressing   ____

     ____

No-cal beverages
(tea, coffee, herb tea, etc.) ____

     ____

Eggs   ____

Peanut butter   ____

Vegetables

Check choice of:

Asparagus   ____

Beets   ____

Broccoli   ____

Carrots   ____

Cauliflower   ____

Celery   ____

Chicory   ____

Chinese cabbage   ____

Cucumbers   ____

Endive   ____

Escarole   ____

Green beans   ____

Green peas   ____

Lettuce	___	Sardines (optional)	___
Parsley	___	Beefsteak and/or	
Radishes	___	hamburger	___
Spinach	___		___
Watercress	___		
Zucchini	___	**Herbs and Spices**	
			___
Meat, Fish, Fowl			___
Chicken	___		
Fish fillets	___	**Other**	
Tuna (canned)	___	(for food preparation)	___
Salmon (canned)	___		___

WEEK 2

Fruit

Grapefruit ____

Apples ____

Bananas ____

Berries (in season) ____

Cantaloupe ____

Pears (optional) ____

Fresh pineapple (optional) ____

Raisins ____

Other (for *safe fruit,*
   fruit salad) ____

____

____

Grains

Whole-wheat bread ____

Whole-wheat crackers
  (low salt) ____

Breakfast cereal (including
  oatmeal) ____

____

Brown (or wild) rice ____

Pasta ____

Dairy Products

Milk (skim or low-fat) ____

____

Cottage cheese ____

Hard cheese ____

Parmesan ____

Yogurt (for Chicken Tomasi) ____

Miscellaneous

Mayonnaise (optional) ____

____

Black olives ____

Chives ____

____

No-cal or lo-cal dressing ____

____

____

No-cal beverages (tea,
  coffee, herb teas, etc.) ____

____

____

Eggs ____

Peanut butter ____

Almonds, slivered ____

Vegetables

Check choice of:

Acorn squash ____

Asparagus ____

Baby onions ____

Beets	____	Other for stir-fry	____
Broccoli	____		____
Carrots	____		
Cauliflower	____	**Meat, Fish, Fowl**	
Celery	____	Chicken	____
Chicory	____	Fish fillets	____
Chinese cabbage	____	Tuna (canned)	____
Cucumbers	____	Salmon (canned, optional)	____
Dark kidney beans (for		Sardines (optional)	____
Mexican Bean Spread)	____	Canned clams, or chopped	
Endive	____	meat (for pasta sauce)	____
Escarole	____		____
Green beans	____	Beefsteak	____
Green peas	____	Beef for pot roast (round,	
Green peppers	____	flank)	____
Lettuce	____	Salmon steaks	____
Mushrooms	____	Pork chops	____
Parsley	____		
Potatoes	____	**Herbs and Spices**	
Radishes	____		____
Spinach	____		____
Tomatoes	____		____
Watercress	____		
Zucchini	____		

SHOPPING LIST FOR MEN'S MENUS

For all three weeks of the Rotation Diet men should use the shopping list of Week 2 for women as their basic list, and check the daily menus to determine what, if any, substitutions they are going to make. There are only a few meals that will require any changes or additions to the basic shopping list of Week 2 for women. These include Eggplant Casserole on Day 12 and a suggestion for Baked Trout on Day 14.

8

APPLYING THE
200-CALORIE SOLUTION
TO DAILY LIFE

I f you make a living at a job that requires sitting almost all of the time, eight hours a day, and if you include only sedentary activity in your leisure time, you are leading an "unnatural" life. The human body was designed to be much more active. When you add a sedentary lifestyle to a diet high in appetite-stimulating supernormal foods, you have the perfect combination of factors that promote obesity.

Most overweight people have trapped themselves in a vicious cycle. The less active they are, the more likely they are to gain weight. The heavier they get, the more uncomfortable it is to be active. As the cycle progresses, physical activity becomes increasingly unpleasant.

The solution is pretty obvious in theory. If you are overweight, you have to eat less or exercise more, or some combination of the two. But in today's world, this turns out to be very difficult to put into practice. I want to deal specifically with the activity side of the solution in this chapter. I'll start with first steps and then move on to suggestions that will help you make an increase in physical activity an integral part of your life.

YOUR OVERALL ACTIVITY GOAL

To begin with, you may feel an increase in your motivation to become more active by facing the facts: if you are a sedentary person, it will be almost impossible to manage your weight without increasing your activity level. And it will help increase your motivation if you realize that *anything* that *reduces* the time you spend in quiet sitting activities and *increases* the time you spend moving about is going to help you toward permanent weight management. These statements are based on the history of the human species.

Up until the advent of the automobile and the availability of cheap electricity, anthropologists and sociologists estimate that humans expended about 500 more calories in energy each day doing their work, maintaining their homes (chopping wood, shoveling coal), caring for their farm or family garden, and transporting themselves to and from wherever they needed to go. During the process of evolution, the human body became adapted to this high level of physical activity, and so did appetites. Until the twentieth century, people in the United States normally ate about 500 calories more each day, and they did not gain weight because they burned up all of those calories in physical work.

Although the need for energy expenditure has decreased significantly in our technologically advanced society, our appetite for food has not. All of the unneeded extra calories are being stored in our expanding fat cells. So how active must you be to stay at your desired weight once you have lost all of the weight you want to lose? I am going to use walking as my first example of an activity, and then relate what I say here to many other examples of exercises later in this chapter (for examples of energy expenditure in various activities, see Table 8-1 on pages 169–71).

Here are the important facts:

Recall that it takes approximately 200 calories to support 25 pounds of fat on the human body. Roughly speaking, walking one mile burns 100 calories. If you walk at what is a comfortable pace for most people (three miles an hour or a mile in twenty minutes), you can burn 200 calories by walking for forty minutes. You can also burn about 200 calories in just thirty minutes once you build up the endurance to walk at four miles per hour.

If you have an excess of 50 pounds of fat in your energy reserves, it has been taking about 400 calories a day to keep your fat cells alive. Thus, it will take eighty minutes of walking at three miles per hour to burn up the 400 calories that has supported the energy needs of your excess fat storage. If you can walk briskly, that is, at four miles per hour, it will take sixty minutes of walking.

Setting a Daily Walking Goal

Before you begin a program to increase your walking, you might find it useful to determine just how much you walk around each day in your normal activities. Most people with a job in which they sit tend to be on their feet and moving around for only about two miles a day. If you use a step counter (and I recommend one that gives you both the number of steps per day and your mileage), you will most likely find that you take only a little over 4000 steps a day. Even if your stride is always 2½ feet long, it takes 2112 steps to equal a mile. Nevertheless, everyone I know who uses a combination pedometer and step counter finds it more rewarding to keep the counter set on number of steps per day rather than distance. Each step you take is rewarding, and you can see your progress in increasing your number of steps each day, or by the minute if you care to.

Dr. James O. Hill,* director of the Center for Human Nutrition at the University of Colorado, suggests that with the use of a step counter, you should gradually increase your number of steps each week until you reach a goal of 10,000. With a stride of 2½ feet, that would total nearly five miles. Thus, if the amount of walking at home and at work each day is just two miles (or about 4000 steps), your goal is to end up with 6000 more steps, or about three miles of extra walking each day.

If you are extremely overweight or simply completely out of condition, you might follow Dr. Hill's suggestion to increase your walking activity by just 500 steps a week (or about a quarter mile). If you are in reasonably good shape and are just 20 to 25 pounds overweight, you may be able to increase your weekly goal and reach 10,000 steps in just three or four weeks. If you have 40 to 50 pounds to lose, you should go more slowly to prevent injury such as back pain and shin splints.

Many people like to think in terms of actual distance or time spent walking, rather than number of steps, since the length of stride can vary greatly throughout the day. So, if you are a beginner in walking for exercise, I suggest you:

1. Walk twenty minutes a day the first week;

* James O. Hill, John C. Peters, with Bonnie T. Jortberg, *The Step Diet* Workman Publishing, 2004.

2. Gradually increase the time until you walk forty minutes a day by the end of the third week;

3. And then increase the time until you walk sixty minutes a day by the end of the fourth week.

If you can do this at a time of day specially devoted to walking, so much the better, since walking as a major daily exercise is an excellent way to increase your physical fitness. If you don't have forty to sixty minutes at a time to walk, the next best thing is to get out of your chair for five minutes on the hour and walk around wherever you are. Eight 5-minute walks will burn about 200 calories.

You will find suggestions for many other ways to integrate more walking and other equivalent energy-burning activities later in this chapter.

When Is the Best Time to Exercise?

The best time to exercise is when it is most convenient. Some people like the energy it gives them if they exercise in the morning; others find it calming to do physical activity later in the day. You can, however, get extra calorie-burning benefits if you engage in some moderate activity after eating. I'll explain why.

It takes energy to digest your food. Normally, it takes about 10 percent of the caloric value of the food you eat to digest it. If you eat 1000 calories, the digestive process will take about 100 calories' worth of energy. However, you can almost double the energy it takes to digest food if you take a walk, *at a moderate pace*, after eating. Thus, instead of using just 100 calories to digest your 1000-calorie meal, you can push it up to almost 200 calories if you go for a twenty-minute walk within an hour after eating.

Consider a walk after your evening meal instead of plopping down to watch TV. It makes a one-mile walk worth almost two miles in number of calories burned in twenty minutes. It can become a pleasant activity for your family or with friends. You will find that as long as you limit exercise in the evening to a moderate intensity, your digestive processes will run more smoothly and you'll even sleep better.

Maintaining Motivation for Walking

Many people who choose walking as part of their weight-management program find it most motivating to make it a social activity. As a pair, or in a group, it is both pleasant and safe. For over forty years my wife, Enid, has been part of a group of women that has varied in size, sometimes as few as five and sometimes as many as nine, who walk early in the morning. They have two routes around a small lake about two miles from our home, and several others in a beautiful park about five miles away. Each route is about three miles long. With a group having that large a membership there are always at least two or three women who will be walking on any given day. The women have a preset schedule of who will be walking each day, and if there is any change in a person's schedule, they let one of the others know.

When you are feeling especially lethargic, and either by preference or by necessity you must walk alone, put on your walking shoes, step outside your door, look around, and take a step or two. Then take two more and you might find your body urging you on your way. Even a short walk around your neighborhood can be refreshing. You might carry tear gas or pepper spray if there are threatening dogs running loose in your neighborhood.

If walking outdoors is not an option, and using a gym is inconvenient, you might find that buying a treadmill for home use is your best option to gain the weight-management benefits of walking.

COMPARISON OF CALORIES BURNED IN DIFFERENT ACTIVITIES

I chose to consider walking first among exercises that help with weight management because for most people walking more is the most convenient and efficient way to increase energy expenditure. For the same amount of perceived effort, walking burns more calories than exercises in which you swing your arms and step in place, as in a calisthenics routine or a beginner's aerobic dance class. While swinging your arms and lifting your legs in one spot may feel like harder work, walking—because you move your entire body weight through space—feels easier than those arm swings and leg lifts, because your body uses your largest muscles (in the buttocks and thighs) for walking, and these muscles are placed in the middle of your body. This placement makes for very efficient movement. In contrast, arm swings use smaller muscles, and the weight that is being moved extends outward from the moving muscles. This is relatively inefficient movement, and it feels harder and is more tiring than walking in spite of the fact that it burns fewer calories.

Swimming is one of the very best exercises for weight management because it requires moving your entire body. Swimming freestyle slowly can burn as many calories as jogging at a five-mile-per-hour pace (that's about 35 percent more calories than a brisk walk, at four miles per hour). Next in weight-management value are **bicycling** (outside or stationary), **elliptical trainers**, and bouncing on a **minitrampoline**. **Ballroom dancing** comes close to expending the same amount of energy as walking at a moderate speed, and **aerobic dance** routines done at a brisk tempo can give you the same benefit as a brisk walk.

Racquet sports are excellent provided you spend most of your time in action, quickly moving around, rather than standing still and socializing. **Tennis** was my daily sport for many years, until I discovered the joys of jogging (which I do not recommend for overweight people). **Racquetball** is easier to learn than tennis, and you tend to burn more calories playing racquetball than tennis in any given period of exercise time. You may want to start off by taking lessons or enrolling in a beginner's class to get yourself started in tennis or racquetball.

Rowing has been eclipsed in popularity by elliptical trainers at my local YMCA. Last time I was there, over four times as many people were on elliptical machines than on rowing machines. Rowing aids in weight management in spite of your not having to move your whole body through space because it uses so many muscle groups throughout your body. Rowing can be a valuable activity for people who cannot do weight-bearing exercise, such as walking, because of injury to their legs or leg joints. However, if you have back problems, discuss the benefits and risks of rowing with your physician. Be sure to start slowly against little resistance until you see how it feels. In fact, you should see your doctor before beginning any exercise program, as well as before starting a diet, as I suggested in Chapter 1.

Later in this chapter I provide more detailed advice for getting started and for equipment needed in some of the activities I have just discussed.

Table 8-1 lists approximate energy expenditure for various activities in a person weighing 154 pounds. Some exercise equipment—for example, elliptical trainers and stationary bicycles—comes with software that enables you to input your exact body weight, and thus may give you a better approximation than the table. You can also learn to use your pulse rate, as I describe in the next section.

Table 8-1 Energy Expenditure in Physical Activities*

Activity	Minutes of Activity					
	5	10	15	30	45	60
Walking						
moderately, 3 miles per hour	22	44	66	132	198	264
briskly, 4 miles per hour	33	66	99	198	297	396
Rebounding†						
brisk walking tempo, little foot lift	22	44	66	132	198	264
jogging tempo, foot lift of 4–6 inches	33	66	99	198	297	396
running, high knee lifts, or kicks	68	136	204	408	612	816
Badminton	34	68	102	204	306	408
Cycling						
leisure, 5.5 miles per hour	22	44	66	132	198	264
leisure, 9.4 miles per hour	35	70	105	210	315	420

Activity	Minutes of Activity					
	5	10	15	30	45	60
Chopping wood						
average tempo	30	60	90	180	270	360
Dancing						
moderate tempo	18	36	54	108	162	216
continuous, intense aerobic	59	118	177	354	531	708
Gymnastics	23	46	69	138	217	276
Horseback riding						
trot, English style	39	78	117	234	351	468
Martial arts, judo, karate						
continuous drill	68	136	204	408	612	816
Rowing						
moderate pace	26	52	78	156	234	312
Running (flat surface)						
a mile in 11½ minutes	47	94	141	282	423	564
a mile in 9 minutes	68	136	204	408	612	816
a mile in 8 minutes	73	146	219	436	655	874
a mile in 7 minutes	81	162	243	486	729	972
a mile in 6 minutes	88	176	264	528	792	1056
a mile in 5½ minutes	101	202	303	606	909	1212
Skiing						
moderate, downhill	42	84	126	252	378	504
cross country	50	100	150	300	450	600
Squash	74	148	222	444	666	888
Stair climbing						
down, rate of 1 step per second	17	34	51	102	153	204
up, rate of 1 step per second	72	144	216	432	648	864
Swimming						
continuous freestyle, slow	45	90	135	270	405	540

Activity	Minutes of Activity					
	5	10	15	30	45	60
continuous freestyle, fast	55	110	165	330	495	660
Table tennis	24	48	72	144	216	288
Tennis						
singles	38	76	114	228	342	456

* Estimates taken from Martin Katahn, *The 200 Calorie Solution*, Norton, 1982. All values are approximate for a person weighing 154 pounds.

† Rebounding exercise moves at a faster pace than walking on a level surface because of the assist given to your movement by the springing action of the minitrampoline.

USING PULSE RATE TO ESTIMATE ENERGY EXPENDITURE AND INCREASE FITNESS

Estimating Energy Expenditure

You can estimate how many calories you burn in various activities that use the large muscles in your body by comparing your pulse rate in those activities with that of walking. Start with taking your pulse while sitting quietly at rest. You can find your pulse just behind your wrist or alongside your neck. Count the beats for fifteen seconds and multiply by four to get your rate in beats per minute (bpm). Then go for a walk at the rate of three miles per hour (for this test, walk at this rate of speed for at least five minutes). Take your pulse again. When you walk at this speed, you will be burning about three times the number of calories you burn while sitting still. On average, this will be about 100 calories per twenty minutes. So your pulse rate while walking at this speed corresponds to burning 100 calories every twenty minutes. Now, if your pulse rate reaches the same rate during other physical activities such as aerobic or ballroom dancing, or moving around on the tennis court, you can feel quite confident that you are getting the same energy expenditure in those activities as in walking at the rate of three miles per hour.

When you reach the point when you can walk briskly (four miles per hour), do this test again. The pulse rate you reach walking at this pace burns about 4½ times the number of calories as sitting still, or about 100 calories in fifteen minutes. You can use this pulse rate to compare with your rate during other physical activities, just as you did with your pulse rate while walking at three miles per hour.

But a word of warning: you should increase the time you walk before trying to increase your pace. When, after a few weeks of walking, you feel ready to increase your speed, do it in intervals. For example, alternate fifty steps at four miles per hour with periods of fifty steps at three miles per hour.

Increasing Cardiovascular Endurance

Your heart is a large muscle, and together with your entire vascular system it gets stronger and more efficient with exercise. To improve cardiovascular endurance, exercise specialists suggest that you walk (or use equivalent exercise) at an intensity that elevates your resting pulse rate by 50 percent. The rate you achieve in this way is called your "target rate." Thus, if your resting rate is 72 bpm, a target rate is 72 + 36, or 108 bpm.* Most overweight

---

* Fitness experts suggest a slightly more complicated way to find your target heart rate that's useful if you wish to pursue higher levels of cardiovascular endurance. Subtract your age from 220. This gives you your approximate maximum heart rate. Beginners should aim for 60 to 70 percent of this figure.

people who are not accustomed to physical activity will reach the target rate walking at three miles per hour. So, as you did to estimate energy expenditure, take your heart rate while at rest and then go out for your walk. If your pulse rate reaches your target rate while you are walking (or doing an equivalent exercise), you can be sure your cardiovascular system is becoming more capable of circulating your oxygen and nutrient-carrying blood throughout your body.

In the WMP we asked participants who were an average of 60 pounds overweight to gradually increase their walking to forty minutes a day and to intersperse brief periods of brisk walking to the extent they could without hurting themselves. Their pulse rate walking at three miles per hour when they began the program averaged 138 bpm (this considerable increase in pulse rate is typical for sedentary obese people). When they were tested walking at three miles per hour at the end of the program twelve weeks later, their pulse rate had decreased to 112 bpm. Thus, within twelve weeks, their heart was working with considerably less effort.

FINDING THE BEST ACTIVITY FOR YOU

While most people find walking to be the most efficient and convenient activity to add to their daily life, you might have some physical activity from earlier in your life that you would like to

---

A person 40 years old would obtain a target rate of 108 (220 − 40 = 180; 180 × 0.6 = 108) just as in the example in the text. Training for higher levels of cardiovascular endurance requires moving up to 70 to 90 percent of your approximate maximum heart rate, which is not at all required for weight management.

restore, or have always wanted to learn. Even if you haven't, you might find hidden in yourself both the talent and great pleasure that can be derived from various kinds of sports, games, dancing, Pilates, yoga, Tai Chi or other martial arts, or strength training. You can find out what activities you might like by joining the YMCA or other fitness clubs, where you can get expert instruction. Many churches also sponsor exercise classes. As many as a thousand members at one of our largest congregations in Nashville get together one time each week to exercise.

In our follow-up each year with participants in the WMP we administered questionnaires, which showed that becoming active is likely to do more for the feeling of well-being and physical self-concept than just losing weight. Since this statement is particularly true for me, I'd like to tell you about the role that physical activity has played in my own successful fight against fat, and the continuing role that it plays in maintaining my health and good spirits. I believe that it holds similar promise for you, if you will only give it a chance.

WHAT PHYSICAL ACTIVITY HAS MEANT TO ME

I learned from personal experience a great deal about what it takes to make physical activity an important part of one's daily life. The very first thing I learned was its value in weight maintenance. I discovered that after losing about 15 pounds during my three weeks of dieting, I could return to my former food intake without gaining weight *provided* I played an hour and a half of singles tennis each day. In my most active days, I needed to consume about

3000 calories a day just to maintain my weight. I can say with a great deal of confidence that *nothing* works like physical activity for weight maintenance.

Without realizing it, however, I stumbled onto another very important key to the success of an activity program: the contribution it made to my self-image. While growing up, my uncle, an expert tennis player, was my childhood idol. I watched him play some of the best tennis players in the country. But he would never agree to give me a tennis lesson. I'm sure he felt that anyone as fat and klutzy as I was could never be a tennis player. While I might have dreamed about becoming a tennis player, I never thought that it was possible either.

My doctor and good friend, Ed Tarpley, changed all of that when he said that I had to become active if I ever wanted to get weight off, keep it off, and help prevent further heart problems. I remembered my uncle and asked Ed if he would approve of tennis. He did, and he gave me the advice to start slowly and moderately.

I began to take tennis lessons and was soon playing singles tennis every day for an hour and a half. Not only did it keep my weight down, but also I began to look forward to those three weeks on my diet because each time I lost 15 pounds I could scamper around the court a great deal faster!

I kept working at my game and improving. Finally, at the end of my first year, I got up the courage to ask one of Nashville's best players to hit with me. This man, Dr. Milt Bush, became one of my closest friends. In addition to being a well-known pharmacology professor at Vanderbilt, Milt was the part-time coach of the Vanderbilt tennis team. He was one of the top players in the United States; at the age of sixty-five, he won both the United

States Grass Courts Championship and the Canadian Open Clay Courts Championship.

One of the things that made Milt such an inspiration was that he won those championships in spite of his having only one arm! If anyone knew what it means to conquer adversity, and to become a champion in spite of it, Milt did. We would meet to hit together, and occasionally he might drop a tennis tip or two. My game began to improve by leaps and bounds.

Soon I began to think of myself as a tennis player. I wasn't playing for the sake of my health anymore, or for the weight-management benefits. These were incidental to the effect tennis was having on the way I thought of myself as a person. People who have never been fat cannot appreciate the thrill former fat persons experience when they discover their hidden physical talents and skills.

Perhaps you, too, had a childhood dream about doing some athletic activity but have felt too embarrassed to talk about it or pursue it. Perhaps you, too, had a secret idol. There is no reason you can't take up tennis, dance, swimming, or any of the other activities I discuss in this chapter when you are older. Many people are returning to such activities or starting for the first time in middle age. I was thirty-five years old when I took my first tennis lesson, and fifty years old when one of my students introduced me to jogging. If being active becomes a part of who you are, as tennis did for me, you can stop worrying about being overweight EVER AGAIN.

Another benefit of becoming active is that it can lead you to find some new, special friends who love the joy of being active, just as I found Milt Bush and my many other tennis buddies. Doing active things together can give you some of the most pleasurable experiences in your daily life.

An Advantage of Exercising Thirty Minutes or More at a Stretch

The steady rhythm of walking, jogging, or swimming can begin to have meditational or hypnagogic effects after about thirty minutes when you do these activities alone, are in a safe place, and can clear your mind of other thoughts by focusing on the steady movement of your body. The refreshing, relaxing, "other-consciousness" effect that can be achieved in this way is so great that yoga masters have, in fact, stated that meditation in motion (as in walking or jogging) is superior to meditation at rest. The so-called runner's high seems to require at least forty-five minutes of a more intense, continuous movement than what walking involves. I have experienced several forms of meditation and relaxation techniques, but once I began jogging, nothing equaled the refreshing, relaxing effects of an hour's gentle jog, alone, along trails in a park near my home. All of the devoted swimmers I know claim the same effects after doing laps in an Olympic-size pool for about half an hour.

HOW EXERCISE CAN INFLUENCE METABOLIC NEEDS

There are two main ways in which you can increase your resting energy needs. Both involve physical activity, and both are important in maintaining weight loss.

On the one hand, by losing weight you reach the desirable goal of having a trimmer, lighter body that takes less effort to engage in physical activities and can make them more enjoyable.

On the other hand, having a smaller, lighter body means it will take less energy to move your body through space, as in walking, and less energy to support all of your basic bodily functions, even while you are asleep or sitting.

If you choose to lose weight by cutting calories alone and remain sedentary, a portion of your weight loss will be in muscle tissue. People who lose tremendous amounts of weight lose some muscle mass because the lighter body does not require as much muscle to move around. Unless you are in that category of overweight, you are better off if you can prevent the loss of muscle mass and even increase it. Here is the scientific reason why.

Muscle tissue is active tissue. In circulating nutrients and regenerating itself, it burns several times the energy of fat tissue even while at rest. Thus, the more muscle tissue lost, the lower your resting energy needs will be.

By increasing your activity to maintain muscle tissue, especially in the major muscles, you maintain those resting energy needs and prevent them from falling even lower than the energy needs of a thinner body. That's why I, along with many other professionals who guide people in weight management, suggest that you add strength training to your daily physical activities. By using light weights, an exercise band, an exercise cycle, doing half squats, practicing getting up and down from a chair, climbing stairs, or using a stepping machine, you may be able to add 2 or 3 pounds of muscle tissue while losing 20 pounds of fat. Note how many of these activities can be done while watching TV or added to daily life, like going up and down the stairs between floors at work or at home. These activities will help maintain your metabolic needs and sustain a weight loss. And these are the kinds of exercise I myself do every day to maintain my muscle mass as I grow older.

They keep me in shape to do most of the things I have done around the house all of my adult life.

There is one other thing you can do to significantly influence your metabolic needs, but only if you are able to lose enough weight to get into condition to exercise vigorously or for long periods of time. Most overweight people, male or female, do not reach this stage of physical fitness. It requires being able to spend at least forty-five to sixty minutes in intense exercise, such as jogging at a speed twice as fast as walking at a moderate speed (a mile every ten minutes instead of a mile every twenty minutes), or taking a hike of several miles. Participating in continuous vigorous aerobic dance for an hour every day would qualify, as would an hour and a half of competitive tennis. Intensive activity at this level for this long can leave your metabolic rate several percentage points higher for an hour or more after exercise. I can remember only three women from one of my own classes in the WMP who went on to become this intensely active and who became athletes for the first time in their lives. Two of them took training courses in aerobic dance and became class leaders at a local fitness center, and another became a marathon runner.

HOW TO BURN EXTRA CALORIES WITH INCIDENTAL ACTIVITY

Over the years that I have been maintaining my original weight loss, I have also been inventing ways to be more active in just about everything I do. During my years as chair of the Psychology Department at Vanderbilt, I never held a meeting in my own office if I could arrange to hold it in someone else's (there was no elevator in the building, so I also had the benefit of walking a few flights of stairs). If it were just a meeting between myself and another member of the department, I would suggest that we go out for a walk and talk. When grocery shopping, as I've mentioned, I always park my car as far from the door to the store as possible (the lack of cars parked next to me also saves my car doors from many dents). Today, as I work at the computer writing, I get up for five minutes of walking around the house on the hour. When I sit reading, I occasionally do a series of leg lifts at the knees or from the hips. A couple of these exercises keep me alert when I'm puzzling over complicated material. While no longer jogging and playing tennis, I do twenty minutes or more on a pedal exerciser twice a day (I can also do this while reading simple stuff or watching the news or a sporting event on TV). I also spend five or ten minutes with an exercise ball, performing exercises especially for arthritis in the lower spinal area. All of these incidental things are in addition to the hour of exercise (which includes fifteen minutes of using light hand weights and exercise to combat arthritis) that I do each morning before breakfast.

I thought I was being quite clever about finding ways to stay active throughout the day until I came across a book by two professors of exercise science and body movement, *The Fidget Factor: The Easy Way to Burn Up to 1000 Extra Calories Every Day* by Drs. Frank I. and Victor L. Katch. The title of the book may be a bit off-putting to people who equate fidgeting with nervousness or restless movements. The book actually contains 159 ways you can add some extra intentional body movement as you perform your daily tasks, such as shifting your weight from one foot to the other as you brush your teeth or as you stand talking on the telephone. Twirling a pencil between your fingers when you sit back to think will burn a few extra calories. One of my favorites, which I have been doing for years, is going up on my toes and down into a half squat while I brew a cup of tea during the day, or wait for the lather to soften my beard before shaving.

Examine what you do each day to which you can add some incidental, nonessential activity at home or at the office. While you may not find it easy to burn 1000 extra calories a day in such activity as with some of the examples in *The Fidget Factor*, you can easily burn an extra 100 to 200 by sitting less and moving more whenever you can, or by just moving any part of your body when you ordinarily would just sit still.

SOME USEFUL INEXPENSIVE EXERCISE EQUIPMENT

There are three pieces of inexpensive exercise equipment that can double or triple your energy expenditure even if you use them only a few minutes at a time during the day.

One of my preferred pieces of equipment is a pedal exerciser, which, as I already mentioned, I use twice a day. You cannot get as intensive exercise with one of these portable pieces as you would on a heavier exercise bicycle, but you can easily double or triple your metabolic rate compared to sitting still. Those sold by Active Living Now (www.activelivingnow.com), Walgreens (www.walgreens.com), and Academy Sports + Outdoors (www .academy.com) are all good. They range in price from twenty-two to fifty dollars. More expensive ones are a little heavier and may come with a timer to help you keep track of the time you pedal. They all take a little experimentation to find the best position for their use. A chair with a sloping back mimics the use of a recumbent bike and a straight-back chair an upright bike. All of the portable cycles seem to work well on either type of chair. They are easy to use while talking at home, watching TV, or listening to music.

A second favorite of mine is a set of rubber exercise bands. Mine come from a local medical-supply store and were prescribed for exercises to combat arthritis and a torn rotator cuff. You can buy Thera-Band Progressive Resistance Exercise Bands at Amazon.com and Active Living Now at reasonable prices. A nearby sporting-goods store may have a set for you to try, to determine the amount of resistance with which you should begin. If you have never done upper-body strengthening exercises, I suggest you start with one or two bands at the lower end of resistance. All you need to double or triple the calorie burning of sitting still is to feel enough resistance to create some strain on your muscles. These bands can be used for both upper- and lower-body strengthening. Five minutes at a time is fine for a break from sedentary activity, but for real exercise you should plan on ten- to fifteen-minute sessions.

I also like using an exercise ball. You can do exercise for your lower back on these balls, as well as lift your legs to mimick marching steps as you sit on it. Marching steps can get an increase in energy expenditure equivalent to a brisk walk in a short time, and tire a normally sedentary person in just a few minutes. The balls vary in diameter from fifty-five to seventy-five centimeters. Mine has a diameter of sixty-five inches and is suitable for people five feet four inches to six feet tall. Choose one that works for your height. Suggestions for exercises for both balls and bands can be found in *Sculpt Your Body with Balls and Bands*, by Denise Austin.

FURTHER SUGGESTIONS FOR SPECIFIC ACTIVITIES

Walking

The most important equipment you need for walking is the right pair of shoes. The problems most overweight participants in the WMP faced were the result of ill-fitting shoes. You need plenty of room in the toe box and about the width of a thumb between your big toe and the end of the shoe. Some beginning walkers experience shin splints if they walk primarily on cement sidewalks or cement floors at local malls. If you plan to walk on cement, be sure to get shock-absorbing shoes or insoles. You will do best by buying your first walking shoes at a shoe store that caters to runners and walkers, where you can try them out in the store and possibly take them home "on approval" for use inside for two days. If you begin to have a problem with your feet or legs when walking a great deal, try a different pair of shoes. If that doesn't work, go to a store that specializes in building customized inserts. Sometimes lower-back problems that develop as a result of walking or standing exercises can be resolved with customized inserts for your shoes.

Swimming

Swimming is an excellent, high-energy-burning activity that is particularly useful for people who have trouble with their feet or ankles while walking. Because of the resistance of the water to your movement, you can burn two to four times the number of calories swimming as you might burn walking the same distance.

Many swimmers tell me that although swimming requires so much more effort than walking, they feel many times better while swimming, and more relaxed physically and mentally afterward.

Swimming and water aerobics are excellent non-weight-bearing activities for overweight people, so I strongly recommend these activities if you prefer to swim or if there are any reasons (for example, arthritis) why you can't walk any length of time.

If you don't feel particularly comfortable in the water, it is well worthwhile to take a few lessons. My wife says she improved dramatically, as did her pleasure while swimming, after reading *Total Immersion*, written by Terry Laughlin with John Delves. Both my wife and daughter swim a quarter to half a mile several times a week at the local Y. But they tell me they often have to wait for a lane. So before you sign up at a swimming facility, you should visit and check out whether the facility is overcrowded at the time that is convenient for you to swim. Also, check to see if they have water classes at a time that is good for you.

A number of women in the WMP told me they were initially embarrassed while shopping for a swimsuit and going to a pool. I can sympathize. It was about six months before I got up the courage to use the university gym to change and shower for my tennis matches on the university courts. I measured fifty-five inches around my hips when I was 75 pounds heavier. I have the stretch marks to show for it, but at thirty-five years I was also young enough for my skin to tighten and avoid very noticeable sagging.

My wife has found a local department store that handles a brand of swimsuit in which she looks best, which saves her a lot of time trying on different suits. After my daughter found the brand and size that suit her best, she began to order her suits online. If you begin to swim, or engage in water aerobics several times a week, you may find that you go through two suits a year, so be sure to have a backup on hand.

Aerobic Dance

Aerobic dancing is a lot of fun and can be done with friends (like other forms of dancing and activities like Tai Chi). Avoid any classes that might involve jumping and leaders who don't allow for a suitable pace for beginners. A good teacher will allow you to adapt exercise to fit your level and any specific problems you have. If the class doesn't suit you, change to another.

At advanced levels, aerobic dance can equal the calorie burning of running at a very good clip. I discovered this for myself at a sports medicine conference. The planning committee had scheduled a two-mile race for one morning, before the meetings began. The doctors who were marathon runners had no problem covering that distance at a five-minute-per-mile pace (as I have said, I am not a fast runner, but I did seven-minute miles that morning for the first and last time). At another session the attendees were given a demonstration of aerobic dance by a well-known teacher and leader of a television aerobics program. She challenged us to participate. Within a few minutes she had the entire group breathing very hard, if not completely out of breath, including the most well-conditioned runners. Aerobic dance involves more upper-body conditioning compared with running, and the runners (and I) were not as well conditioned for it.

Strength Training

I have already discussed the importance of maintaining your muscle mass as you lose weight. If you have a great deal of weight to lose, for example, 50 pounds or more, it's quite likely that you will lose some muscle in your legs.

People who do not engage in some kind of aerobic activity or strength training can lose so much muscle mass as they age that they might experience a reduction in metabolic rates by as much as 5 percent per decade. Some may lose as much as 20 pounds of muscle by the time they are sixty-five years old. You can restore part of that loss with strength training no matter how old you are.

I have used light dumbbells to maintain upper-body strength and exercise bands for both upper- and lower-body strength for many years. I was not trying to bulk up, so I used lighter weights and did more repetitions. You can use heavier dumbbells and do fewer repetitions if you want to gain larger muscles. However, I want to reassure women worried about looking bulky that doing light strengthening with three- to five-pound dumbbells and exercise bands in the lower range of resistance will just make you look trim. Because you can run the risk of dropping a dumbbell if you use one for exercise, you might consider using them while you are on a floor mat, or in bed for that matter! As for all exercise, ask your doctor or an exercise specialist at your gym for advice on using free weights and other strength-training apparatus.

Flexibility Exercises

For general gentle flexibility exercises, I recommend the exercises that you can find in the book *Arthritis: What Exercises Work*, by

Dava Sobel and Arthur C. Klein. The book covers exactly the exercises my physical therapist recommended for me to combat my arthritis. They are just as useful for helping anyone maintain flexibility, and especially useful for anyone who already is experiencing back pain. I wish that I had started doing these exercises before I began to develop arthritis in the lumbar region of my back several years ago.

For all kinds of stretching exercises suitable for various sports and for specific activities such as traveling and gardening, and for folks with physical limitations or working at the computer, take a look at *Stretching: 30th Anniversary Edition*, written by Bob Anderson and illustrated by Jean Anderson. You can find more details about the book online.

In the next chapter, I show you, with the help of your new, more active lifestyle, how to increase your food intake without regaining any of the weight you lost on the Rotation Diet.

9

TAKING A VACATION
FROM DIETING

The Transition to Maintenance

Why do you have to stop now and take a vacation from dieting? If you have more weight to lose, why can't you just continue using the Rotation Diet over and over again until you lose all the weight you need to lose?

If you have reached your goal weight, why do you have to make a "transition" to maintenance? If you haven't lowered your daily energy needs beyond what is to be expected for a lighter body, why can't you begin your celebration immediately and eat anything you want?

Let's start with why you need to take a break in dieting. First, a break in dieting guarantees that your metabolic rate will not slow down, which is likely to occur when you use a very-low-calorie diet for too long.

Second, the break increases your motivation to be as perfect as possible during each three-week period that you are on the Rotation Diet. Longer periods of dieting can encourage small deviations, followed by larger deviations, finished off by complete collapse.

Third, if you have problems controlling your appetite, you are not as likely to begin to overeat after only three weeks of dieting as you are if you had forced yourself to endure several more weeks or months of deprivation. Long periods of dieting can build up powerful hidden impulses to binge.

Fourth, you need the practice of maintaining small weight losses on your way to complete success. It is much easier to manage maintenance after three separate 10- or 15-pound losses than it is to manage your weight after losing 30 to 45 pounds all at once. With each 10- or 15-pound loss you discover what you need to do with your diet and activity program to stay at your new weight, and you begin to incorporate the metabolic benefits that go with increased physical activity and improvement in your diet. In previous chapters, you learned some of the things you need to do to maintain or even increase your total daily metabolic needs. Later in this chapter, I discuss some additional metabolic benefits that you can obtain from improving the quality of your daily diet.

Now, to address the other questions, we need to start with water retention. Because "water retention" is blamed for any number of things when weight fluctuates, you need to understand the way water balance varies in your body, apparently whimsically (but really lawfully), increasing and decreasing its total water content while still tending to hover around some central point. A number of factors are involved in causing these fluctuations, and they can all come into play and affect your weight.

Even if your weight has generally been stable for a period of time, you have probably noticed how it tends to jump around within a range of about 2 pounds over a one- to three-day period (or even 4 or 5 pounds if you weigh 200 pounds or more). For example, you go out to a party on a Saturday evening and have a couple of glasses of wine, some snack food, perhaps a rich main course, and then dessert. You wake up pounds heavier the next morning. In order to gain a true 2 pounds of weight in fat, you would have had to eat about 7000 calories more than your normal intake. (Each pound of body fat contains about 3500 calories.) You know darn well you haven't binged to that extent. You may have had 1000 extra calories, but certainly not 7000. How can you gain 2 pounds on 1000 calories?

Now take the opposite situation. It's the middle of the week, you haven't been on a reducing diet, you haven't been around any desserts or alcohol, and you have been too busy to cook anything except simple food. Perhaps, in addition, you ran out of salty snacks. Over a three-day period you may have eaten 500 calories a day less than you did over the last weekend. Now, on Thursday morning, you find yourself 2 pounds lighter than you were on Monday. What accounts for this?

As I indicated, it's a question of water balance.

The human body is, on average, about 72 percent water. This means that a person weighing about 140 pounds has a body that contains about 100 pounds of water. Muscle tissue, for example, is 75 to 80 percent water, blood is almost 100 percent water, and the sugar energy stores in the liver (glycogen) are dissolved in a ratio of one part sugar to three or four parts water. In addition, there is a considerable amount of fluid all around the body cells. Thus, given 100 pounds or more of water in our bodies, it is easy to imagine that there are many different factors that might cause water content in the body to vary by 2 to 3 percent (2 to 3 pounds) in a few days, or even overnight.

SOME FACTORS AFFECTING
WATER BALANCE

Sodium

Excess sodium can cause a major amount of water retention when we take in more than our kidneys can dispose of quickly. There is enough sodium in just one medium-size pickle to cause a 1-pound weight gain in susceptible people. Similarly, if you have what is essentially a low-calorie Chinese meal, you can show a 2- or 3-pound weight gain the next morning without having overeaten by one single calorie. The gain is primarily due to the sodium in the MSG and, possibly, to the overuse of soy sauce. For this reason, and because many people are allergic to MSG, many Chinese restaurants will make your food without MSG.

Changes in Calorie Intake

Although you might be aware of the effects of too much sodium on your body weight, you might not understand how an increase *of only 500 calories* in one day can also lead to a 1-pound weight gain. The body responds to a change in caloric intake much as it would to a dose of sodium. You can gain weight at about 1 pound for each 500 calories beyond your daily energy expenditure, up to a total of about 2000 calories more than your usual intake (at which point the body's ability to store more water purely due to caloric overload would stop).

Most people give themselves a double whammy when they go off the deep end and begin to overeat. They combine an increase in sodium consumption with an increase in calories. If you over-eat by 500 calories each day for three days (or stuff in 1500 extra calories in one day), and fail to watch your sodium intake, you can easily gain several pounds. This sort of weight gain is especially likely to happen to sedentary people because they do not do any-thing in the way of physical activity that can get rid of some water via perspiration and respiratory activity.

You can see the most dramatic illustration of rebound water retention (technically called "the rehydration effect") after people have been on a complete fast in order to lose weight. I was once invited to visit a medically supervised fasting program. While there, I observed obese men who had just finished three weeks of fasting gain 7 pounds in five days on a diet *of only 600 calories per day!* Since the average loss for the group was 20 pounds, this meant they were regaining weight faster than they had lost it.

GUIDELINES FOR MAKING A SUCCESSFUL TRANSITION TO MAINTENANCE

In order to prevent a rebound weight gain after being on the Rota-tion Diet for three weeks, you must follow certain rules. You can-not immediately binge to celebrate all the weight you have lost, and you can never return to a sedentary lifestyle (assuming you have increased your activity level) without endangering your weight. You are obliged to keep burning up, on a daily basis, all of the calories it used to take to maintain your former excess weight, to prevent the fat you've lost from creeping back into your fat cells.

Increase Food Intake Slowly

Of all the guidelines, this is probably the most important. If you increase food intake too quickly, you will probably increase both calories *and* sodium.

For those of you who have followed my cold-turkey method for three weeks, I suggest not adding more than one serving of any of the supernormal foods you may have eliminated from your diet (for example, fried food, various combinations of sugar and fat in desserts, and salt in snacks) until you check your weight the next day to see its impact. By not rushing back to consuming any of the high-calorie foods that contributed to your being overweight, you might find that you actually lose another pound or two.

If you have just completed the twenty-one days of the Rotation Diet by following the meals and menus I have suggested, do not increase your food intake to more than 1200 calories each of the next three days if you are a woman, and 1800 calories a day if you are a man. To make the transition to maintenance as easy as possible, women can use the 1200-calorie menus of Week 2 again (page 90), and men the 1800-calorie menus (page 97). *If you want to be absolutely sure you will not gain weight, use the Week 2 menus for a whole week.* When participants in the WMP used the Week 2 menus for a full week in transition, they often lost 1 or 2 more pounds.

After women have been on the 1200-calorie menus for three to seven days, they should increase their intake to 1500 calories and stick with 1500 calories for three days, using the 1500-calorie menus that I have laid out for men (pages 94–97, and pages 249–52 in the Alternate Menus in Chapter 11). Do not add more than one serving of a supernormal food on any given day until you check your weight the next day to determine its impact. With daily moderate activity for an hour (or brisk activity for forty-five minutes), women should be able to reach a daily intake of between 1800 and 2000 calories sometime during the fifth week after beginning the Rotation Diet. Being able to reach a caloric intake at this level requires forty-five to sixty minutes of physical activity. Use my 1800-calorie menus as guides (pages 97–100, and pages 253–58 in the Alternate Menus). After spending three to seven days on 1800 calories, men also go up by 300-calorie increments, first to 2100 calories for three days, and then to 2400 calories.

You can, if you like, consider this week your "vacation from dieting" and start all over again the next week. But I always took at least a month off between rotations, and you may be happier and more successful if you do the same. It can give you practice in maintenance and keep your motivation at a peak level.

A good strategy during your entire transition to maintenance is to think in terms of 300-calorie increments until you determine where your weight will stabilize with your new level of physical activity. Since we are all different, it is necessarily a testing process.

For those of you who don't wish to follow my menus, and for men going up to 2100 and 2400 calories, I would suggest, to be on the safe side, adding only extra servings of fruits, vegetables, and lean meat, fowl, or fish to meet the 300-calorie increases. You can build your own menus using my recipes, since these recipes will give you the calorie contents for each serving. For other foods, see Appendix A for calorie, fat, and fiber estimates. In general, note the following:

Except for *free vegetables*, half-cup servings of vegetables will contain around 25 calories.

The average-size piece of fruit will run around 60 calories, with small fruits (such as a plum) containing around 40 calories and large fruits (a large apple) containing about 80 calories.

You can consider *lean meats*, fish, and fowl to contain about 55 calories per ounce, and you will not be far from correct. But watch out for the fat! Fatty meats can run over 100 calories per ounce.

Avoid Excess Salt

After consuming a bowl of onion soup, a couple of tablespoons of blue-cheese dressing or a couple of pickles to go with a salami sandwich, you may find yourself a few pounds heavier the next morning. In order to prevent these extra pounds, cook with a minimum of salt or cut it out entirely. You will use much less salt if you add it to taste at the table. That's because the salt grains on the surface of food meet your taste buds first and "leap out at you." And learn to use herbs and spices as I suggest in my many recipes.

Following is a list of foods high in sodium. Eliminate those that have no nutritional value and eat in moderation those that do. For example, be moderate in your consumption of most cheeses. They are an important source of calcium, but they also tend to be high in sodium (compare package labels). Avoid foods that contain not much more than just sodium and fat (for example, bacon and sausage). Purchase the low-sodium or no-sodium-added version of a food if it has one.

anchovies and anchovy paste
bacon

baked beans with pork

baking powder

beef, corned, dried

bouillon cubes (except low sodium; check label)

canned vegetables (except low salt or salt free)

celery salt (plain celery seed is fine)

cereals (check label; the best ones will have less than 250
milligrams per serving)

cheese (blue, cheddar, processed)

corn, popped with salt added (okay plain)

crab, canned (salt can be reduced by about half by washing
and draining)

crackers, soda type

fish, smoked and salted

ham

ketchup in large quantities

olives

peanuts, salted (unsalted in the shell are recommended)

pickles

potato chips and other similarly salted snacks

pretzels (unsalted okay)

processed luncheon meats, including vegetarian substitutes

saltine crackers (reduced salt okay)

sauerkraut

sausage

soups, canned (reduced salt or no salt added okay)

soy sauce (reduced-sodium variety in small amounts okay)

TV dinners (check labels, most are very high in sodium)

Worcestershire sauce

Eat Naturally Diuretic Foods

Some foods have a natural diuretic function. They stimulate your kidneys to rid your body of water, rather than close them down as do the salty foods just listed. Naturally diuretic foods tend to be relatively high in potassium content, compared with their sodium content.

Here is a list of foods that will help you get rid of excess water. The most effective ones seem to be fresh pineapple, asparagus, citrus fruits, and green vegetables.

apricot
asparagus
banana
beef, lean
broccoli
cantaloupe
chicken
cottage cheese (low sodium)
figs
grapefruit and grapefruit juice
lamb, trimmed
milk, skim and low fat
nuts, unsalted
orange and orange juice
pineapple, fresh
potato
prune and prune juice
raisins

tomato
tuna, water packed
turkey
watermelon

Be Physically Active

Almost as important as the fat-burning power of physical activity is its aid in preventing water retention. Normally, on any given day, we lose almost as much water through perspiration and respiration as we do through the kidneys. (Our breath is 100 percent saturated with moisture when we exhale.) When we are active, we can lose 1 to several pounds of water through perspiration, and as we increase our breathing rate, we can double the loss of moisture through respiration. *You can retain a couple of pounds of water on any day that you skip your activity session.* So it is absolutely essential that you maintain your activity level during the transition to weight maintenance.

Drink a Glass of Water before Meals

Drinking a glass of water before meals is a proven strategy that helps prevent overeating. In fact, so does having a bowl of low-fat, low-sodium soup. Adequate fluid intake stimulates the kidneys and helps to reduce water retention, and your body has to burn some calories in the process. In addition, adequate water intake will keep you regular and prevent the gain of a pound or two of refuse weight. Also, substituting water in place of the dietetic beverages you might have used in the past will help prevent the reawakening of your sweet tooth!

Remember Your Safe Fruit

Perhaps the two most important dietary changes that have stayed with me in all my years of weight maintenance have been the elimination of all fried food, and the substitution of fruit, fresh and dried, as snacks and desserts, for salty, high-fat snacks and junk foods.

You, too, will find weight maintenance a snap if you substitute fresh or dried fruit for most of your previous snack foods and for a good part of your desserts. Use low-fat frozen yogurt to replace ice cream, and instead of commercially baked desserts, try some of the recipes in the Alternate Menus chapter in this book. Many of the dessert recipes in cookbooks will still taste great if you cut by one-fourth to one-half the amount of fat and sugar called for.

There you have it. I know that you have worked hard to lose the weight you have lost. Having been on the yo-yo myself during the first thirty-five years of my life, before I found out how to maintain my own weight loss, I know how frustrating it can be to let your weight start creeping up again. Follow my guidelines to make a transition to maintenance, and you, too, will achieve permanent weight control. Here they are, once again, in summary form:

1. **Increase Food Intake Slowly**
2. **Avoid Salt and Salty Foods**
3. **Eat Naturally Diuretic Foods**
4. **Be Physically Active on a Daily Basis**
5. **Have a Glass of Water (or a Bowl of Low-Fat, Low-Salt Soup) before Meals**
6. **Make Fruit Your Substitute for Junk Food in Your Diet**

Now we are ready to discuss the two permanent weight-management benefits that you can obtain by making one very significant change in the quality of your diet.

KEEPING THE FAT OUT OF YOUR FAT CELLS

It is much easier to gain weight from overeating fat than from overeating carbohydrate or protein. Per gram, fat contains 9 calories, while carbohydrate and protein contain just 4.

But there is also another factor that makes it easier to gain weight from fat than from carbohydrate or protein. Fat is easily converted to a form that your body can use for energy, and it's very easy to convert dietary fat to body fat for storage. It is especially easy to gain weight if you happen to eat more fat than your daily energy requirements.

Carbohydrate and protein require more digestive work to convert their energy for direct use in bodily processes than does fat, and this results in a "wasting" of some of the energy. That is, some of the calories are burned up and thrown off as heat.

Similarly, if you overeat either carbohydrate or protein, the body has to work considerably harder to change these nutrients into fat storage than it does to change dietary fat into fat stores. It takes between four and five times more energy to convert carbohydrate and protein to fat than to convert dietary fat to body fat.

Perhaps this will become intuitively evident if you just imagine a quantity equal to two teaspoons of fat or oil sitting in a dish next to a fairly large apple. Both food items will be approximately equal in calories (70 to 80 calories). However, your body will have to work a lot harder to change the calories in the apple (should you even be able to overeat fresh apples) into body fat than it has to work to change the calories in the fat or oil into body fat.

It takes about 5 percent of the energy content of dietary fat to convert it to body fat. It takes 20 to 25 percent of the energy in carbohydrate and protein to turn these nutrients into body fat.

So, besides the fewer calories per gram in both carbohydrate and protein compared with fat, the additional energy needed to do the metabolic work involved in its direct use and storage is another reason for limiting fat and basing your diet primarily on carbohydrate and protein foods.

An Increase in Dietary Fiber Helps in Weight Management

Two other factors prevent weight gain when you increase the amount of *complex* carbohydrates (whole grains, fruits, and vegetables) in your diet and decrease fats.

First, foods with complex carbohydrates, and only these foods, contain dietary fiber. Fiber is included in the calorie counts in your calorie books, but the body doesn't digest these calories! Our stomachs and intestines don't have the appropriate enzymes to break down that fiber (other animals do). So, depending on the particular carbohydrate foods you eat, perhaps 10 percent or even more of the total number of listed calories passes right through your system with the roughage.

Second, as an extra metabolic benefit, the fiber contained in the complex carbohydrates will attach to about 10 percent of the dietary fat you eat, and that, too, will pass right through your system without being digested.

So, can you, in fact, "increase your energy needs through eating"? If you substitute complex carbohydrates for fats in your diet, the answer is yes. If you cut your fat consumption in half and instead start eating fresh fruits and vegetables and whole-grain products, you may find that you need a much larger volume of food than you are presently eating, just to get enough calories to maintain your present body weight.

MOVING ON

In this chapter, I explained the details of how you can make a transition to maintenance that will keep off the weight you lost with the Rotation Diet. If you have more weight to lose, after a week's or a month's vacation from dieting (it's up to you), go back on the diet.

Now, in the next chapter I show you how to meet the lifelong challenge of *permanent* weight management.

10

WEIGHT MAINTENANCE

A Lifetime Challenge

n the opening chapter of this book I asked, "If people can lose weight so quickly and easily on the Rotation Diet, why bother to update and revise it?"

I answered that question by saying, "It's one thing to lose the weight. It's quite another to keep it off." Keeping weight off is a lifetime challenge. I want to go into detail here about how I and others are able to do it.

The challenges we face require that we learn to deal with a supernormal-food environment that encourages overeating. Not only are our supermarkets brimming with processed foods scientifically designed to overstimulate our appetites, but also restaurants are competing with one another, touting bargain prices for supersized portions. As I turned on the TV to watch the news recently, a sit-down restaurant chain advertised a dinner for two for $14.99, with choice of barbequed ribs or deep-fried shrimp, French fries, and choice of another side dish. In the next commercial break, a fast-food chain advertised a double cheeseburger so thick the actress in the ad could barely open her mouth wide enough to take a bite.

THE NATIONAL WEIGHT
CONTROL REGISTRY

We can get a good idea what strategies successful people use to achieve and maintain weight loss from the National Weight Control Registry (NWCR). The NWCR is a database of folks (now around 5000 registrants) who have lost at least 30 pounds and have kept it off for at least a year. The founders of the registry, Dr. James O. Hill, director of the Center for Human Nutrition at the University of Colorado and Dr. Rena Wing, professor of psychiatry and human behavior at Brown University, and their colleagues, have published their findings in a number of studies. You can access these studies at www.nwcr.ws. Once you have lost at least 30 pounds and kept it off for a year, you too can join the registry. With the help of Dr. Hill, I have spoken with some of the registrants in the NWCR, and I believe that membership helps them maintain motivation to continue using the strategies that led to success. Here is a summary of the NWCR findings. I encourage you to visit the website for the titles and abstracts of the principle research articles.

About 90 percent of the participants took more than one attempt to lose weight and keep it off. The only common characteristic was that 89 percent of the successful participants used both diet and exercise to lose weight. Only 10 percent used diet alone, and just 1 percent used exercise alone. I believe the reliance on both diet and physical activity is important since most weight-loss programs put the main emphasis on diet, while physical activity is at least equally as important in maintenance.

People in the registry used many different approaches to dieting to lose weight, and no single approach stood out. When they finally did succeed, it was in a way that they designed for themselves to fit their life situations. About 75 percent of the registrants began their last diet because of a serious health problem or a traumatic life event such as a divorce. About 55 percent of the registrants lost weight by participating in a formal weight-loss program, while 45 percent did it on their own.

While participants used various approaches to lose weight, there are four behaviors in common among them for maintenance:

1. Eating a low-fat, high-carbohydrate diet;
2. Having breakfast almost every day;
3. Frequent monitoring of their weight;
4. Engaging in a high level of physical activity.

Participants reported eating a diet rich in fruits and vegetables, with fat comprising 23 to 24 percent of daily calories. This corresponds very closely to the diet we suggested to maintenance participants in the WMP, which contained about 25 percent of calories in fat. The average American diet contains between 35 and 40 percent of calories in fat. A truly low-fat diet would contain about 15 percent in fat. Cutting back to 25 percent of calories in fat is a rather modest change, but it works.

About half of the participants count either calories, fat grams, or both. Some pay primary attention to portion size, while others cut out particular foods or whole classes of foods (like fried foods, cake, or candy).

Some participants weigh themselves at least once a week; others every day. It's a question of what works best on a personal basis. Some people avoid the scale because they are afraid of what they will see. Others use what they see to make adjustments in food intake and exercise to make sure they stay closer to their lower weight. They set a limit to a weight gain of, say, 3 pounds over their desired base and then take corrective action.

Participants in the NWCR reported that, on average, they devoted eighty minutes a day to planned physical activity. The most preferred activity was walking, but many added high-intensity activities like aerobic dance and strength training. The average calorie expenditure devoted to physical activity for women was about 2500 calories a week, and for men about 3300 calories a week. (For women, that's about the equivalent of twenty-five miles of moderately paced walking each week and for men about thirty-three miles a week.)

When I have mentioned this finding to folks over the years (the initial findings of the registry came out in the late 1990s), most have responded with either disbelief or thought, "I can't do that. Even if I wanted to, I don't have time." However, once a person becomes committed to daily activity of this kind, it strengthens the motivation to maintain the other aspects of the maintenance program. When we interviewed people in our follow-up research in the WMP, they would often say they were not going to eat in a way that would waste the calorie-burning effort they had put into their daily exercise.

MOTIVATION

This research doesn't tell us the most important things we need to know: *Why* do successful people continue to do what it takes to keep their weight off? What is the payoff in following a lower-fat diet? *Why* do they exercise? *Why* and *how* do they deal with the established habits and circumstances in their lives that led them to become overweight? I'll talk first about the challenges we face in becoming more active.

In my own case, I was about as sedentary a person as one could be when I weighed 230 pounds back in 1963. I would put off climbing even one flight of stairs if I could avoid it. My health problems, high blood pressure and a heart attack, provided the initial motivation to lose weight. Things like these are "push" factors. It's a little like running away from wild animals. They get you started. What most people miss in developing a lifelong maintenance program is the "pull" factor. They don't find anything in their lives that "pulls" them to behave in ways that have greater value than what they can put in their mouths! For me, the pull factor was the payoff in enjoying tennis and jogging, and becoming good at them.

I have always considered physical activity to be a key to permanent weight management. It is at least as important as, if not more important than, dietary discipline after a goal weight has been achieved. But the sad truth is that the majority of overweight people who start an activity program fail to reach and maintain the daily goals they originally set for themselves.

I believe that the deciding factors in whether a person becomes and *remains* an active person are psychological and emotional. The greatest motivation to become and remain an active person is to find some activity that contributes to your self-image, builds your self-esteem, and ends up making you feel good, just as tennis and jogging did for me. If you choose an activity that requires special skill, strength, or endurance, you must participate in it enough so that you see yourself improving. The better you get, the stronger your motivation to continue will become.

SUCESS STORIES

Participants in the NWCR Tell Me
about Themselves

When I spoke with participants in the NWCR, they told me what motivated them to lose weight, how they dieted, and why they continue to include activity as part of their weight-management strategy. With permission I taped our conversations and here are some excerpts. (I have not used their real names.)

BONNIE

I spoke with Bonnie when she was forty-six years old. She told me that she was thirty-eight and weighed 235 when she got serious about losing weight. It began with her mother nagging her, as she had often done, to join a commercial weight-loss program. But Bonnie was a registered nurse employed at a local hospital, and program meetings would not fit well into her frequently changing work schedule.

One night when she was on duty, the call light went on several times simultaneously from two patients. She had to hurry up and down a long hallway to reach them. At one point she arrived at a patient completely out of breath and embarrassed. She said to me, "You know, when you are going to take care of people, you don't want a nurse huffing and puffing when she comes up to take care of you."

This started a chain of thought. She began to think of her future. She said, "You know, I'm also a single person [she was divorced the year before she began her weight-loss regimen], and I'm by myself, so I have to take care of myself."

Bonnie took three years to lose 65 pounds because she found it difficult to adhere to any caloric reduction for very long. She said she would just cut back on portions, and added, "But I think the basic thing that really, really helped me was that I got into exercise. I bought a used alpine climber from a girlfriend, like a StairMaster, and I can honestly tell you that the first time I got on it, it was just for two minutes, and I thought I was going to die. I just kept working at it every night I'd come home. And I'm now at the point I can do forty minutes solid!"

Bonnie went on to tell me that over the years she began to incorporate Richard Simmons tapes because she likes to do aerobics to music, and that she tapes TV shows to watch while she is on her climber. She added 5-pound weights to her exercise because "my arms were getting flabby."

However, Bonnie's weight does fluctuate quite a bit. She said she has never quit eating sweets and never quit eating desserts. Near the start of our conversation she said, "Today I actually had dessert and I couldn't believe it, because I need to lose 5 pounds. But I thought this is my day off and tonight I will not eat that much. I'll probably cook a pork chop or something on the grill and have a salad—something light." Then she said that when she does eat big meals, she compensates with extra exercise when she gets home at night. It reminded me of what a participant in the WMP once said to me: "When I split a dessert after dinner, it means 20 extra minutes on the treadmill." I call this the "penitence" method of weight control. I don't knock this method when it is followed religiously. For many successful people, it serves as the fallback method of choice for preventing their regaining the weight they have lost.

TRACY

I spoke with Tracy when she was forty-five, four years after her husband had left her. During the year that followed his leaving, she lost 130 pounds at the rate of about 10 pounds a month by eliminating fried food, fast-food burgers, butter on her baked potatoes (which she is now very fond of eating with salsa or chives), and almost all bread. When I spoke with her, she said she was keeping her weight in a range between 122 and 125 pounds. She also told me, "The one thing that I still have problems with—I walk past a window and see my reflection and I have to do a double-take because I still don't believe it's me. I still see a fat Tracy in there and I have a problem with that. But I love buying clothes!"

She started walking about nine months after beginning her diet and became what she called "an avid walker," covering two miles every day and more on Sundays. "I was religious on that. I had my time to walk, and I enjoyed it, and it didn't matter if it was 110 degrees or if it was 40." She also told me that she had joined a step-aerobics class, but she had recently given it up due to a bad car accident in which she had hurt her back and shoulders. At the time I talked with her, her physical therapist had okayed stair climbing and walking again, so she had become a member of a group of four women at the company where she works, and together they climb fourteen flights every day. She reserves walking for weekends.

KATHERINE

Katherine is thirty-three years old. She lost 55 pounds in a fourteen-week period three years before our conversation. She followed a strict very-low-calorie diet of her own design, focusing on lean meat, fruits, and vegetables and omitting bread ("bread is my downfall") but including small portions of rice or potato. She said she thought she consumed about 700 calories a day during the entire period. (Most people underestimate the caloric value of their diets, but Katherine averaged a weight loss of almost 4 pounds a week. I doubt, however, that she actually consumed only 700 calories a day, since, as you will see, she began to greatly increase her exercise to the point where I think she would not have been able to take in so few calories and still do her daily job, take care of family responsibilities, and begin her exercise program. Nevertheless, however many calories she actually ate, it certainly worked.)

She told me that while both her parents are overweight, she did not actually gain weight until she reached twenty, and gradually came close to weighing 190 pounds. She became particularly concerned when she reached thirty and recalled that her mother had had three heart attacks in quick succession at age thirty-two. "I didn't want to have that—I have four small children and I wanted to get the weight off before I turned thirty-five."

Together with her strict diet, Katherine started working out from week one. "I started at three half-hour workouts a week at a club—a twenty-four-hour workout place. I found a workout partner. I work in the same salon with Donna. She was going to her gym and I was going to my gym and I said, 'Why don't we just start going to this one and go together?' So we started going to classes together, then we started doing weights together, then we started doing elliptical trainers, and it was really nice because it's on the days when you say to yourself, 'I really don't want to go,' Donna announces, 'I'm ready.' It was extremely helpful."

Katherine's workouts went from an hour and a half a week to ten hours a week.

She now goes for two hours, five times a week. While her main job is as a hair stylist, a year ago she took a part-time job at the gym as an instructor. Almost everyone where she works at her primary job was "very, very neat about the whole thing," but two were "a little bit envious." They "tried to play sabotage," bringing food into work and teasing her for not eating. "Overall, I'd say 98 percent were incredible. My husband is ecstatic. He loves it. He loves it that I feel so good."

Katherine has a collection of before and after photos and enjoys showing them. People who didn't know her before she lost weight are amazed at the change because she is not recognizable as the same person from the before photos. One of her friends who knew her before she began her weight-loss program, and then saw her again after she had lost 55 pounds, exclaimed, "Now you're a bombshell."

Two More Recent Successes

Normally I never initiate a discussion about weight with anyone. But as I was writing this chapter I broke my rule and asked two acquaintances who lost significant amounts of weight in the last three years to tell me how they did it and what they are doing to keep it off.

LISA

Lisa is a professor at a Nashville university. After asking her one afternoon to tell me how she lost 40 pounds, she sent me the following email in which she alternates between giving advice and telling about herself. While my views don't always correspond with hers, they work for her.

Here are Lisa's twenty rules for permanent weight management:

1. Start by weighing yourself. I have an old-fashioned doctor's scale, and it's very reinforcing to move the little weight down, if even by a half millimeter, every morning. Weigh first thing every morning, same time. Keep a chart of weight loss to document your progress.

2. Set a goal—know your body mass index, and aim for the normal range. I started by trying to lose 2 pounds each week, then after the first loss (which comes quickly), 1½ pounds, then 1 pound each week. As you lose weight you will feel good about yourself every morning as you slide that weight ever lower on the scale. You will have more energy and your clothes will fit better. All great reinforcers to keep on track.

3. You learn to like what you eat. If you eat healthy, you crave healthy.

4. Don't buy junk food (potato chips, for example, I love them) or fattening foods (vanilla ice cream for me). Throw them out if they are in your pantry. If they are not there, when you get hungry you won't turn to them.

5. The first week is the hardest because you will be hungry. Eat, then leave the kitchen—even if you are still hungry, it will pass after half an hour. And your stomach does shrink over time and you do fill up with less food. [Your stomach probably does not shrink, but you will most likely feel satisfied with less food in your belly.]

6. Eat vegetables. Learn to love them. But if you eat salads, watch the salad dressings. If you are still hungry after you've eaten what's on your plate, have another helping of vegetables.

7. Have some stock foods that are filling that you love and that are good for you. I get a whole-wheat, multigrain bread I love at Costco. I slice it very thin, toast it, and put almond butter on it after I come home from swimming (when I'm always famished). It does the trick.

8. Or eat a banana; it's filling and good for you.

9. I also drink freshly squeezed grapefruit juice in the morning, a large glass. It tastes wonderful and has the enzymes to process the sugars.

10. KEEP MOVING. If you exercise for an hour each day, preferably in the morning, your metabolism is jacked up the rest of the day. You have more energy and burn more calories. Best to have two reasons for exercising: first because it makes you healthy and increases weight loss; second reason is, for me, social pressure. Meeting friends to go walking, swimming with your husband—these work for me.

11. Drink water. It cleanses the body and uses up some of those consumed calories because it has to be heated to body temperature and excreted by the kidneys.

12. Get enough sleep. People who don't sleep enough put on weight.

13. Fresh is best. If it has a store shelf life of longer than a week, don't buy it. It's full of preservatives and corn syrup. Read the ingredients label before you buy.

14. Milk products are fattening. Substitute lentils, beans, vegetables—a little low-fat milk is okay, but no cream for sure, and also no cheese, which is high in animal fat. [Cheese and low-fat yogurt remain a part of my own diet and a significant source of calcium for me.]

15. No desserts. If you stop eating them you will stop craving them. Remember, a moment on the lips, forever on the hips.

16. No soda drinks. They are either full of sugar with no nutritive value, or they have aspartame or other nasty sweeteners that are really bad for you. [Aspartame and other artificial sweeteners are generally recognized as safe by the FDA, but I don't use them, either.]

17. No pizza—it's VERY fattening, full of fat, salt, and empty carbs.

18. I don't crave alcohol, so it's easy for me to skip it. It's converted by the liver to sugar, adding unwanted calories to the dieter.

19. Avoid eating out or getting take-out food. These meals are almost always high in salt (retention of water), fat, and sugar. And, because you've paid for the food and the portions are usually huge, you feel compelled to eat everything. There goes the diet. [I have some suggestions for eating out in Chapter 6 and elsewhere.]

20. When you hit certain goals (first 10 pounds, for example), reward yourself with a new piece of clothing that shows off your new figure.

RHONDA

Rhonda is a thirty-year-old Egyptian immigrant who came to the United States a few years ago. When her second child was born in 2009, she planned to nurse him, but her job at a local manufacturing plant soon made it impossible. One day she announced to me and several friends, "I know how to lose weight," with no further information. I didn't ask for any either—not then, nor a short time later when she came in looking exactly as she did before becoming pregnant. She had lost 22 pounds in the two months after she had stopped nursing her baby.

When I was gathering information for this book, I asked Rhonda to tell me how she lost her weight. She went over each meal, telling me that she ate the same thing every day.

For breakfast she would have a piece of hard bread that she bought at a local Egyptian grocery (it sounded to me like biscotti) that she could dip into hot cocoa (made with milk). She added a small piece of cheese.

For lunch she had a big salad that she brought to work every day. It had plenty of lettuce, plus some tomato, cucumber, celery, and onion, seasoned with a little bit of salt and a tablespoonful of vinegar (no oil). She also had a piece of bread (except for the biscotti-like bread for breakfast, she bakes her own) and two slices of "boiled" meat. I believe she meant braised, but she emphasized no fat and no butter. She always simmered her meat before adding any vegetables for a stew, and then continued cooking it for another hour. And she emphasized, "Green tea every time."

She was finished with lunch by two in the afternoon. Between two and five o'clock she would have a banana, or an orange, or "a lot of watermelon." She said she never ate anything after five.

Rhonda now works as a packing clerk at a local department store. She moves around twelve hours a day in a cubical with a conveyor belt on either side. There are shelves front and rear, which hold the packing materials and boxes for everything from shoes to small appliances. She often has to go up one to three steps on a small ladder to reach these materials. Merchandise comes in on her right, and leaves after she packages it on her left. She works 20 percent faster than is required, to earn bonuses for exceeding the quota required for all workers, which, as you will see, impacts the amount of exercise she gets.

I told her I was curious about how many steps she took each day, explaining that some experts said that a person needed to take 10,000 steps a day to help make sure they do not gain weight after dieting. I gave her a step counter to wear, and she called me the next day to say that she hit 9500 steps at work the day before—and did some housework when she got home, to hit 10,000. Between the work in which she earns half the family income, and her work at home, where she cooks, cleans, bakes bread, and raises two children, she expends about the same amount of energy it would have taken a woman living 125 years ago in the United States to take care of the family home and vegetable garden.

My primary purpose in including this group of success stories is to give you a broad picture of the overall plans these different people have used. Now I want to go more into depth about dietary issues.

THE DIETARY CHALLENGE

I have already explained how I was able to eat whatever I wanted during the years I was most active. It was a time when I expended about 1000 extra calories each day in the activities I had grown to love. Katherine, in her story above, is one of the few women to equal this kind of energy expenditure. Like myself she was in her thirties when she began her weight-management program. As a teenager she was of average weight and had taken dancing lessons, so she knew what it was like to be thinner and active. She had something already in her memory to look forward to.

Many overweight people are not going to have the time and opportunity, even if they have the desire, to be as active as Katherine and I became. Most people in sedentary jobs, even if they integrate two miles of walking each day (which burns about 200 calories) into their routine, will probably find they can easily out-eat that daily extra energy expenditure. If you are likely to remain a person with limited time or ability to expend more than 200 calories a day in physical activity and are or have been more than 25 pounds overweight, it is of even greater importance that you learn deal with a supernormal-food environment.

Understanding in vivid detail how the American food environment is actually designed by the food industry to entice us to overeat can add to your motivation to take control of the situation yourself. I suggest you read *The End of Overeating*, by Dr. David A. Kessler, a former commissioner of the Food and Drug Administration. You may see yourself in the book, as I did. It is also available on CD.

In the story of Andrew that Dr. Kessler presents, I saw myself as I was forty-eight years ago. Andrew is a forty-year-old man, about five feet nine inches tall and weighing about 245 pounds. Forty-eight years ago I was five feet ten inches tall and weighed 230 pounds. Andrew finds his out-of-control-eating behavior repulsive. He loathes himself for his inability to control his appetite. Pizza and M&Ms are irresistible. Each day is a struggle, as it once was for me. I thought of my favorite pizza toppings when I was a fat man: double cheese, vegetables, chopped black olives, and anchovies. Two of my other favorite dishes were potato salad and chopped chicken liver (it didn't matter whether the liver was made with chicken fat or mayonnaise). I could eat a pint of chopped liver at one sitting. I recalled how, as a teenager, I would sneak down into the kitchen at night, slice a couple of pieces of bakery rye or pumpernickel bread, lather them with mayonnaise, and make a thick sweet onion sandwich. Andrew's obsession with food was so realistic a description of my own relationship with food in bygone years that I began to get extremely uncomfortable, actually nauseated, listening to it. I turned off the CD! There is no way in the world I could ever again be involved with food in such a destructive way.

Dr. Kessler is not particularly optimistic about anyone's ability to control overeating once it has been learned and become habitual in response to highly palatable foods and the stimuli associated with them. He believes we need to recognize overeating "as a chronic problem that needs to be managed, not one that can be fully cured."

Yet, some people *are* cured. I am—or have been for almost five decades! So is Katherine, at least for the past three years. But Dr. Kessler is right insofar as much of the research literature is concerned. Most people don't reach the weight-loss goal they desire, and after losing whatever they do achieve, they often lapse. The ones who recover from their lapses and get back on track have developed backup strategies to reinstitute control and prevent complete collapse.

It's up to you to decide just how hard you are willing to work to change your eating behavior. It's going to take determination, backed by a strong drive to implement a plan of action to break old habits and establish new ones. But that is the lifelong challenge all of us face if we truly desire permanent weight management.

FUNDAMENTALS

Whether you are reading this before beginning your first rotation on the diet or while making your transition to a weight-maintenance diet, you might find it helpful to learn what your food intake is really like for a week.

If you include in your diet any of what I have called supernormal foods, such as fried foods, high-fat snack foods like chips and cheddar-cheese crackers, desserts like cake and pie, candy, and other salt, fat, and sugar combination foods, you will likely find it revealing to keep an eating diary. You can do this in a small spiral-bound notebook that fits easily into a purse or shirt pocket. Remember to mention everything in the diary, including a handful of nuts or a single piece of chocolate. A great deal of useful information can be culled simply from the number of times during a day or during a week that you eat any foods from the categories that are mainly responsible for promoting obesity. To be more exact, you might list the time and portion size. You can get even more precise by weighing and measuring your food for a week or two, as we trained participants to do in the WMP. That is most likely to be useful if you decide that you wish to control portion size and include more than an occasional supernormal food in your maintenance diet.

Interestingly, when we showed new participants in the WMP how to keep an eating diary and asked them to keep a baseline record for a week of "normal eating" before starting a reduced-calorie diet, over a quarter of the women in the group had the largest single week's weight loss in the entire ten-week program, and they supposedly weren't even making an effort to lose weight!

Just keeping track is often enough to deter people from choosing foods they know contribute to being overweight, and encourages them to make better choices.

Many successful weight losers continue to keep diaries of what they eat. About half keep track of the number of fat grams, or calories, or both. If you want to be at all scientific about it, I suggest you pick up a copy of the *DietMinder: Personal Food and Fitness Journal* published by MemoryMinder Journals. This journal lets you keep a good record of what you eat all day, including the amount of calories, fat, carbohydrate, fiber, and protein. There's a column to add another nutrient of your choice. It's laid out so that you can also track your intake of vitamins, supplements, and medications, as well as your physical activity, on a daily basis. A section containing "Favorite Food Facts" is in alphabetical order to help you find the nutritional information you might need to fill out the daily diary.

BREAKING OLD HABITS AND MAKING NEW ONES

There are both external and internal cues that can set off an eating response. Obviously the sight and smell of food, together with the anticipation of a very pleasant taste, can stimulate your appetite, but so can the thought of eating and the past association of food as a response to stress, frustration, anger, and other emotions. Let's start with the external cues.

If you wish to change your behavior in the presence of food, you need to break the chain of events that takes place between the sensory response to the food and the neural impulse that sends your hand reaching for it and placing it in your mouth. Simply put, you have to extinguish a well-established pleasurable bad habit and replace it with a better habit.

Learning to do this can take several steps. It begins with generating new thoughts or ideas about food that take the place of old ones and inhibit signals from the part of your brain that turns on your appetite. This is followed by rehearsal, practice, and the use of fantasy or imagination until new habits are firmly established. (An example follows below.) The new habits cannot be felt as a cross to bear for the rest of your life. You have to remind yourself of the payoff in a slimmer body so you know it's worth doing.

Problem Areas

I'm going to cover several areas, including resisting temptation, managing eating in social situations, and making poor food choices. But first, you need to think about the quality of your diet and your eating habits.

Just about all people who have lost a significant amount of weight and are successful in keeping it off classify foods as either good or bad. They also think of their eating behavior as either good or bad. Sometimes the categories are as clear as black and white in their minds. Other people think of both their behavior and different foods along a continuum of good and bad. Sometimes they *almost* completely eliminate certain foods from their diets, but they occasionally do consume a bad food. When they do, they have practiced making it the result of a conscious decision, not an impulse, and have established strategies that prevent regaining any of the weight they have lost.

Here are examples of two "resisting temptation" problems. The first, while it is quite easy to deal with, is unavoidable.

NIBBLING WHILE PREPARING MEALS

You are preparing a tasty, full-course dinner. All of the dishes you are preparing are good foods. The problem is how to keep yourself from nibbling on snack foods and prevent yourself from numerous unnecessary taste-testings while you are cooking. Consider some of the possible strategies.

You can keep a toothpick in your mouth or chew gum. Some people wear surgical masks every time they cook a tempting dinner! These tactics don't require a great deal of planning or practice. If you decide on one of these approaches, have the material (gum, toothpicks, surgical mask) on hand, and just do it!

Or you can nibble on *free vegetables*. I began to use this solution after cutting back on salt in my diet. In the past, nibbling on free vegetables while I was preparing a tasty dinner was not very satisfying. A celery stalk without a stuffing of cream cheese or peanut butter held no attraction for me. But after drastically cutting my salt intake several years ago, my sensitivity to the flavor of unsalted vegetables increased greatly. I discovered how the flavor of each bunch of celery and carrots differs, and how sweet they are without salt. The same is true of different-color bell peppers. Since I like to prepare the vegetables for our evening salads, I now cut up bite-size pieces of celery, carrots, and bell peppers and set them to the side as I begin to make the salad. In this way, instead of being concerned about snacking while preparing dinner, I get another serving of nutritious "free" foods several times a week.

CONTROLLING YOUR RESPONSE TO SUPERNORMAL FOODS

Most people who are successful in dealing with supernormal foods keep them out of the house. This is not always possible if you live with other people. Your job is to learn how to turn off your attraction to these foods, which is pretty hard for most people. Some people keep supernormal foods in their diet, learning portion size to control the amount they eat at any one time. However, lapses are common. When this happens, they put into practice the behaviors that will get them back on track.

The following suggestions are based on the instructions I used and the role playing we practiced in WMP groups. The procedure is designed to break an existing uncontrolled, unhealthy response to specific foods. After the habit is broken and conscious control is established, it may be possible for some people to return such foods to their diet to a limited extent.

In my groups, I would put a bar of chocolate on the table at the front of the room to act as an example of a supernormal food. To get the most out of the tactics and overall strategy of this exercise, you should set the stage by putting a supernormal food you like right in front of you.

1. To eliminate an established undesirable reaction to such foods, you have to first stop dead in your tracks and immediately begin a substitute combination of thought and action. You can't just leave yourself hanging there in a kind of vacuum. So, while staring at the bar of chocolate, shout to yourself (silently or out loud if you are alone), "STOP! THIS IS A KILLER!" Some people use the phrase, "This is poison." The phrases represent the fact that the food might actually shorten your life by its effects on your health as well as your weight. ("Thought stopping" is a proven technique in cognitive behavior therapy that gives you greater control over behaviors you want to change.)

2. Continue this line of thought. Get your dander up over the fact that when you see and then eat this food, your behavior is controlled by "demonic" food scientists. Knowing the kinds of flavors humans are attracted to, they have created super-delicious foods that have you behaving like Pavlov's dog and that can take control of your appetite center. These scientists are not demons, of course. It's their job to create foods that will augment the industry's bottom line (the damage to your "bottom" line is just collateral damage).

3. Continue to use your imagination in developing a course of action other than eating. In role playing, one member of the group would offer the chocolate to another, who practiced the "No, thanks" response. So imagine that you are with another person who is offering you something in the supernormal category. You might continue with, "Not right now; another time," or simply, "No, thanks." The "No, thanks" response can save you a lot of dietary grief. It is well worth practicing in the examples that follow.

4. It's also helpful to express your determination to change your reaction to the food by turning your back to the display. Stand still for a moment, review your memory for what you have just done, and give yourself credit for having taken a step to put your eating behavior under better control.

This exercise can also be done by having a better choice of food available, such as a piece of fruit on display next to the supernormal food. You can then make the act of choosing a part of your practice. But it's useful to do it with the supernormal food alone, since your being offered it without a healthful alternative is harder to deal with. That's when you pull out a simple "No, thanks."

The Great Usefulness of Fantasy, Imagination, and Mental Rehearsal

Before going on to some other steps to be taken in different situations, I want to encourage you to use fantasy and imagination in plotting the changes you want to make in your eating and activity behavior. Many people don't realize how important it can be to use them and mental rehearsal in building successful performance in many areas of life. Seeing yourself clearly in your imagination carrying out every step in detail helps assure a good, if not perfect, performance.

Having given many concerts in my first career as a violinist, and having become a pretty fair tennis player at a later age, I know the mental work it takes to build self-confidence and then test your ability in front of others. Actors, musicians, and champion athletes all visualize themselves on the set, the stage, or the field performing their challenge. This mental activity is an essential part of practice, just as essential as the physical part. Playing out success in your mind helps to block an anticipation of failure, which can become a self-fulfilling prophecy. You may feel this way when it comes to weight management—you expect failure and you get it!

Let me emphasize that *attention to specific behaviors* is very important in mental rehearsal. For example, tennis players put their effort into visualizing perfect strokes and a plan of attack. They spend little time dreaming of the trophy! Many people attempting to use fantasy as an aid for change make the mistake of dreaming about the end product, when they should be concentrating on the *means* to that end. When I was a violinist, it was one thing to dream about being a success on the stage, but I soon learned that the most profitable time had to be spent mentally rehearsing the bowings and fingerings of the selection I was to perform, and hearing the music inside my head as I watched the score flow by my closed eyes. Working mentally with attention to detail, I was able to increase my comfort on stage and my technical skill.

You, too, can apply a productive fantasy to plot your strategy for weight management. You may also find that doing it while on a walk gives you an uninterrupted opportunity to make plans in this and other areas of your life.

ADDITIONAL EXAMPLES

Here are other situations and examples in which the use of fantasy, imagination, rehearsal, and actual practice can help you become your own best problem-solver.

To resist the temptation of eating at home, it's good to have in reserve an activity that is incompatible with having food in your hands. Knitting or crocheting is excellent for this purpose, but so is playing a game of cards or a musical instrument, setting up a chessboard to work on a problem, or getting someone to play a board game.

There's something about watching TV in the evening that inspires eating, even after a big dinner. Changing your behavior when everyone else in the family is eating some fattening food while watching TV takes a lot of practice. If the urge to eat is strong, use your mental practice to substitute a food like fruit, low-salt/low-fat crackers, or air-blown popcorn. Watching TV is also a good time to use a pedal exerciser.

Social situations are difficult for maintaining weight. At buffets for large gatherings of people, survey the selection of food, pick out the most healthful dishes, and retire to an area far from the food table. Don't finish all of the food on your plate, so that if the host comes around to offer more of something, you can point to your plate and say, "I'm still working on this."

It is worth setting up a practice situation at home. Put a single piece of food that you might find at a party, for example, a piece of cheese, on a small plate. Place the plate on a cocktail table or your lap and imagine a host approaching you with a tray of goodies. Then point to it as you look up, and say, "No, thanks. Not right now." Use whatever expression you like to courteously decline the food you wish to avoid.

Similarly, making a good choice from a lengthy restaurant menu can be difficult. Many formerly overweight people put up a kind of *Star Trek* shield when they enter a restaurant. Dr. James Hill, when talking about how successful members of the NWCR deal with food choice in restaurants, calls it a "portable mini-environment" into which only the "good foods" can enter. Once you have decided what foods fit into your diet and how you like them prepared, you will find yourself doing this too. Don't be shy about asking for foods to be prepared according to your criteria if you don't see anything on the menu that fills the bill.

When it comes to *overeating*, many people working to reform their eating habits give up when they make the first deviation from their eating vows. If you ever say or think of a self-defeating expression like "I just can't resist (name a food)," that expression has to be eliminated from your vocabulary. Never, never use it again. You *can* learn to resist. Yes, it is possible to *begin* to overeat, and *still stop yourself.* Work through the familiar fantasy steps that you have used for other eating-problem areas: imagine yourself beginning to overeat, stopping yourself, and returning to your rehearsed eating plan. It does become easier with practice.

One of the best rehearsal strategies *for learning* to deal with overeating is to buy a food item in a single portion that frequently tempts you to overeat, and set up a situation in which you can eat it slowly and with pleasure. Be sure to allow up to twenty minutes for observing yourself and your reactions after you finish eating, so that you can see how your appetite begins to turn off and how the urge to continue eating disappears. Then store the image of the experience in your memory so you can draw on it as needed.

Why does the urge wane? Eating for twenty minutes allows enough nutrients to be absorbed so that signals begin to reach the appetite centers in the brain. I reformed my habit of eating quickly by surreptitiously watching a slow eater and matching my pace to his.

A NOTE ON JUNK FOOD

One definition of a junk food is that it supplies, per serving, a greater percentage of the calories necessary to maintain body weight than it does the percentage of the Recommended Dietary Allowance of even one essential vitamin or mineral, or of the daily recommendation for fiber.

The easiest way to check on the nutritional status of a processed food is to check the label on the packaging. With 2000 calories as the average daily quota to maintain weight, 100 calories is 5 percent of a day's need. Thus, if you find no vitamin, mineral, or fiber content at least equal to 5 percent of the RDA on the food label, it's a junk food, and you should seriously consider how much of such foods you want in your diet.

Really nutritious foods that you can use as snacks, such as *safe fruits*, have a much higher percentage of essential vitamins and minerals than they do of weight-maintenance calories. For example, 100 calories' worth of pink grapefruit contains 7 percent of the RDA for iron, 22 percent of vitamin A, 12 percent of thiamine, 5 percent of riboflavin, 5 percent of niacin, 192 percent of vitamin C, and about 14 percent of potassium. And since grapefruit contains virtually no sodium, the high potassium content makes it an excellent food for people who tend to retain water or are interested in controlling their blood pressure. (Before eating grapefruit, check with your physician if you are on any medication, since grapefruit can interact with a number of different drugs.)

EATING AND THE EMOTIONS

There is a complex relationship between food and pleasure centers in the brain. Eating supernormal foods can cause the release of hormones that help blunt the experience of strong negative emotions. Thus, eating "comfort foods" like chocolate or salty snacks can become an unfortunate way of dealing with stress, anxiety, or anger for many people. So, for the lack of better options, comfort foods can lead to overeating and overweight.

If there are circumstances in a person's life associated with the weight problem (as sometimes happens when folks fall into unfortunate relationships and working situations they hate), the best solution is to deal with those circumstances directly and make changes when they are necessary. Trusted family members or friends are often the first places people turn to for assistance. For those with a religious affiliation, some congregations have an experienced counselor as well as a pastor or priest to help. As a final resort, it may be necessary to enlist the help of a professional therapist.

But for just about all of us, life presents situations that create tension, even when we have excellent personal relationships and a job we love. Physical activity can be a great stress reducer and a great way to think through issues. The practice of Tai Chi reduces tension, improves balance and flexibility, and provides an efficient way to burn calories. While joining a class is probably the best way to learn Tai Chi, I recommend any of the DVDs made by Dr. Paul Lam for home study, including: *Tai Chi for Older Adults; Tai Chi: 6 Forms 6 Easy Lessons*; and *Tai Chi: The 24 Forms.*

Other palliative ways to help clear your mind and deal with stressful situations include meditation and deep muscle relaxation. There are a large variety of instructional CDs on these practices. Two meditation CDs that I especially like are *Walking Meditation* by Nguyen Anh-Huong and Thich Nhat Hanh, and *Guided Meditations* led by Bodhipaksa.

If you suffer from high blood pressure in addition to stress, you may find it helpful to use a RESPeRATE, a battery-operated electronic device that, with a pleasant sound track, can train you in slow, relaxed breathing. Check this out at www.resperate.com. This device can be used effectively to reduce tension regardless of whether or not you have high blood pressure.

The next chapter contains Alternate Menus and recipes to add variety to further use of the Rotation Diet.

11

ALTERNATE MENUS FOR THE ROTATION DIET

The Alternate Menus include a number of new recipes created by my wife, Enid, and our daughter, Reyna—everything from soups and salads to main courses and desserts, as well as styles of cooking from around the world.

You can choose a complete day from the Alternate Menus to substitute for any equivalent day in the standard menus on the Rotation Diet. Just make sure you are at the appropriate calorie level. I include Alternate Menus for each level of the Rotation Diet, from 600 to 1800 calories.

If you do not like sticking with any full day in its entirety, you can mix and match your own meals. The calories are listed for all of the recipes in this chapter as they were for the standard recipes in Chapter 7. Choose a standard breakfast at each level, if you like, and repeat it for several days if that will make your food choice easier. (If you choose a fortified cereal for breakfast, such as 40% Bran Flakes or Raisin Bran, you will help ensure that the nutritional value of your diet closely approximates the Recommended Dietary Allowances, even at 600 calories per day.)

For lunch and dinner, however, be sure to include a wide variety of different foods both during your twenty-one days on the Rotation Diet and in maintenance.

If you design your own menus at any time during the Rotation Diet, remember the formula:

women   *For Weeks 1 and 3:*
          600 calories for three days
          900 calories for four days
          For Week 2:
          1200 calories for one week

men   *For Weeks 1 and 3:*
          1200 calories for three days
          1500 calories for four days
          For Week 2:
          1800 calories for one week

MAINTENANCE

Women

The 1500- and 1800-calorie menus in this chapter are perfect for women as you build up to your maintenance intake after the Rotation Diet. Try them to ensure that you do not regain any weight. You can alternate these menus, or substitute them, for the 1500- and 1800-calorie-per-day menus that I suggest for men in Chapter 7. If you wish to follow your own inclinations on your way to maintenance, be sure to increase by only 300 calories per day, and stick with 1500 for several days before going up to 1800.

Men

On entering maintenance, men should also remember to increase from 1800 calories per day, up to your maintenance levels, in amounts of about 300 calories per day. Be sure to stay with 2100 calories per day for several days, checking your weight, before moving up to 2400. It is best to increase your calories with fruits, vegetables, whole grains, and lean meats, but you can try a serving of a dessert or alcoholic beverage if you like. Check my quick calorie guide in Appendix A to make sure you do not increase by too much too rapidly.

Everyone

Remember that *free vegetables* and your *safe fruit* are available at all times, and that a substitution of fruit of any kind for junk-food snacks will go a long way toward preventing weight gain after you have used the Rotation Diet to reach your goal.

MEAL PREPARATION WITH THE ALTERNATE MENUS

Any of the dishes marked by an asterisk in the Alternate Menus that follow will have a recipe in this chapter, right after the daily menu plans. Some of the dishes from the standard menus have been included, so if you do not see an asterisk after a dish in the Alternate Menus, be sure to check the index or go directly to Chapter 7 to find some cooking suggestions. If you follow your own inclinations, remember to prepare food in a plain fashion, without added fat or sugar, except as permitted in each rotation.

All weights in the following menus are cooked weights. The calorie counts in the recipes allow for shrinkage due to cooking.

600-Calorie Rotation

MENU 1

BREAKFAST
½ grapefruit
½ cup of oatmeal
½ teaspoon of cinnamon
4 ounces of skim milk
Coffee or tea

LUNCH
1 cup of bouillon
Open-faced sandwich: 1 slice of whole-grain bread,
1 ounce of lean meat, and Dijon mustard
Unlimited free vegetables
No-Cal Salad Dressing
½ cup of peach slices
4 ounces of skim milk
No-cal beverage

DINNER
2 ounces of skinless chicken breast, oven-broiled
Fresh spinach salad
No-Cal Salad Dressing
½ cup of brown rice
No-cal beverage

MENU 2

BREAKFAST
8 ounces of plain yogurt
1 cup of berries, sliced
1 slice of whole-grain toast
Coffee or tea

LUNCH
Chef salad: add 1 ounce of turkey, carrots, bell
peppers, celery, and unlimited free vegetables
No-Cal Salad Dressing
5 whole-wheat crackers
No-cal beverage

DINNER
1 cup of red beans
½ cup of brown rice
2 tablespoons of grated cheese
½ cup of cauliflower
½ grapefruit
No-cal beverage

MENU 3

BREAKFAST

Cheese toast: 1 ounce of cheese and
1 slice of whole-grain bread
1 orange
Coffee or tea

LUNCH

Tomato stuffed with ¼ cup of shrimp or tuna
1 cup of tossed salad
No-Cal Salad Dressing
5 whole-wheat crackers
1 apple
No-cal beverage

DINNER

Egg Drop Soup*
Turkey and sprout sandwich: open-faced with 1 slice
of whole-grain bread, 1 ounce of turkey, and Dijon
mustard
¼ cantaloupe
No-cal beverage

900-Calorie Rotation

MENU 1

BREAKFAST

1 low-fat Whole-Wheat Breakfast Cake*
2 tablespoons of maple syrup
8 ounces of skim milk
Choice of fruit
Coffee or tea

LUNCH

2 ounces of Baked Chicken
1 cup of Spinach Salad
No-Cal or Lo-Cal Salad Dressing
½ cup of fresh fruit
No-cal beverage

DINNER

3 ounces of Seafood Italia*
½ cup of cooked carrots
1 side-dish serving of Succotash*
1 baked potato
1 teaspoon of butter or 2 teaspoons of sour cream
No-cal beverage

MENU 2

BREAKFAST

8 ounces of skim milk
½ cup of hot cereal
½ teaspoon of cinnamon
2 tablespoons of raisins
Coffee or tea

LUNCH

Cup of soup (your choice)
Open-faced sandwich: 1 slice of whole-grain bread
with 2 ounces of lean meat, sliced tomato,
and Dijon mustard
1 cup of lettuce salad with carrots, celery, and
cucumber
No-Cal or Lo-Cal Salad Dressing
½ grapefruit
No-cal beverage

DINNER

2 ounces of Chicken Sesame*
¾ cup of brown rice
¾ cup of yellow squash
1 cup of fresh fruit
No-cal beverage

MENU 3

BREAKFAST
1 ounce of dry cereal
4 ounces of skim milk
1 orange
Coffee or tea

LUNCH
4 ounces of Medley Casserole*
1 serving of Vegetable Soup with Barley*
4 ounces of skim milk
½ grapefruit
No-cal beverage

DINNER
3 ounces of Paprika Pork Goulash*
½ cup of noodles
1 cup of broccoli
1 pear or peach
No-cal beverage

MENU 4

BREAKFAST
½ cup of cooked cereal
2 tablespoons of raisins
8 ounces of skim milk
Coffee or tea

LUNCH
1 cup of bouillon
1 serving of Salmon Loaf*
1 cup of tossed salad
No-Cal or Lo-Cal Salad Dressing
5 whole-wheat crackers
1 apple
No-cal beverage

DINNER
1 serving of Mrs. Dash Country Chicken and
Mushrooms*
1 baked potato
1 teaspoon of butter or 2 teaspoons of sour cream
½ cup of cauliflower
1 cup of berries and melon balls
No-cal beverage

1200-Calorie Rotation

Remember that when you reach the 1200-calorie level, or above, you may add 1 tablespoon of butter, oil, or other fat within the calorie guidelines. You may also add 3 *safe fruits* within the calorie guidelines.

MENU 1

BREAKFAST
8 ounces of skim milk
½ banana
1¼ cup of dry cereal
Coffee or tea

LUNCH
1 cup of salad: lettuce, tomato, radish, green pepper
Lo-Cal Salad Dressing
6 whole-wheat crackers
8 ounces of plain yogurt
1 cup of berries
No-cal beverage

DINNER
4 ounces of Baked Fish in Spring Herbs*
1 cup of Oven-Fried Potatoes*
1 cup of cooked cabbage
1 apple
No-cal beverage

MENU 2

BREAKFAST
8 ounces of skim milk
½ cup of oatmeal with cinnamon
2 tablespoons of raisins
1 slice of whole-grain toast
Coffee or tea

LUNCH
1 cup of Broccoli-Cauliflower Soup*
5 whole-wheat crackers
1 ounce of cheddar cheese
1 cup of tossed salad
Lo-Cal Salad Dressing
½ grapefruit
No-cal beverage

DINNER
1 serving of Shrimp and Snow Peas*
1 cup of steamed asparagus
1 cup of fresh fruit
1 slice of whole-grain bread
No-cal beverage

MENU 3

BREAKFAST

8 ounces of plain yogurt

1 cup of berries and melon balls

1 slice of whole-wheat toast

Coffee or tea

LUNCH

12 ounces of Mushroom Clam Chowder*

1 cup of Seasoned Tomato Salad*

4 Toasted Oat Thins*

½ grapefruit

No-cal beverage

DINNER

4 ounces of Halibut Steak with Vegetables*

1 cup of Citrus Carrots*

¾ cup of Peas and Baby Onions

1 cup of sliced peaches

No-cal beverage

MENU 4

BREAKFAST
8 ounces of skim milk
1 low-fat Whole-Wheat Breakfast Cake*
2 tablespoons of maple syrup
½ banana
Coffee or tea

LUNCH
1 cup of Egg Drop Soup*
Chicken and Swiss Salad*
½ melon
No-cal beverage

DINNER
4 ounces of Spicy Orange Pork*
1 side-dish serving of Succotash*
½ cup of brown rice
½ cup of unsweetened applesauce
1 cup of tossed greens
Lo-Cal Salad Dressing
No-cal beverage

MENU 5

BREAKFAST
8 ounces of skim milk
1 German Fruit Puff*
Coffee or tea

LUNCH
1 serving of Curried Lentils*
Unlimited free vegetables
Lo-Cal Salad Dressing
6 whole-wheat crackers
1 pear
No-cal beverage

DINNER
4 ounces of Chicken Teriyaki*
1 serving of Chinese Fried Rice*
1 cup of steamed zucchini
1 serving of Pineapple Ice*
No-cal beverage

MENU 6

BREAKFAST
8 ounces of skim milk
1 slice of whole-wheat toast
1 teaspoon of preserves
1 orange
Coffee or tea

LUNCH
1 cup of soup (your choice)
2 slices of whole-grain bread
2 ounces of chicken
Unlimited free vegetables
Lo-Cal Salad Dressing
½ melon
No-cal beverage

DINNER
4 ounces of lean broiled beefsteak
1 cup of brown rice
1 cup of green beans
1 cup of peach slices
No-cal beverage

MENU 7

BREAKFAST
4 ounces of skim milk
1 bagel
½ grapefruit
Coffee or tea

LUNCH
Turkey and sprout sandwich: open-faced with 1 slice
of whole-grain bread, 1 ounce of turkey, and Dijon
mustard
1 cup of Spinach Caesar Salad*
1 banana
1 cup of bouillon
No-cal beverage

DINNER
1 serving of Mrs. Dash Crunchy Popcorn Chicken*
1 cup of Spicy Green Beans*
1 small baked potato
1 serving of Bread Pudding*
No-cal beverage

1500-Calorie Rotation

MENU 1

BREAKFAST
8 ounces of skim or low-fat milk
1 cup of hot cereal
2 tablespoons of raisins
4 ounces of grapefruit juice
Coffee or tea

LUNCH
1 serving of Salmon with Dill*
Unlimited free vegetables
Lo-Cal Salad Dressing
5 whole-wheat crackers
1 apple
No-cal beverage

DINNER
1 Artichoke-Stuffed Portobello*
1 cup of steamed broccoli
1 serving of Polenta*
1 Apple-Nut Bran Square*
No-cal beverage

MENU 2

BREAKFAST
1½ ounces of dry cereal
1 banana
8 ounces of skim or low-fat milk
Coffee or tea

LUNCH
¾ cup of cottage cheese
6 whole-wheat crackers
1 cup of steamed cauliflower
½ melon
No-cal beverage

DINNER
12 ounces of Shrimp Jambalaya*
1 cup of cooked green beans
1 cup of cooked carrots
5 whole-wheat crackers
1 serving of Bread Pudding*
No-cal beverage

MENU 3

BREAKFAST
8 ounces of plain yogurt
1 cup of berries
1 slice of whole-wheat toast
Coffee or tea

LUNCH
1 cup of soup (your choice)
2 slices of whole-grain bread
¼ cup of Tuna Salad
Unlimited free vegetables
Lo-Cal Salad Dressing
1 banana
No-cal beverage

DINNER
One-fourth Lean and Perfect Pizza*
1½ cups of tossed salad
Lo-Cal Salad Dressing
1 cup of fruit
No-cal beverage

MENU 4

BREAKFAST

8 ounces of skim or low-fat milk
1 German Fruit Puff*
Coffee or tea

LUNCH

4 ounces of Quick Skillet*
1 cup of tossed greens
Lo-Cal Salad Dressing
1 apple
No-cal beverage

DINNER

4 ounces of Halibut Steak with Vegetables*
1 cup of Stovetop Spinach Casserole*
1 small baked potato
1 slice of whole-grain bread
1 piece of fruit
No-cal beverage

1800-Calorie Rotation

MENU 1

BREAKFAST
8 ounces of skim or low-fat milk
1 poached egg
2 slices of whole-wheat toast
1 teaspoon of preserves
½ grapefruit
Coffee or tea

LUNCH
6 ounces of Chicken Paprika*
1 cup of Potato Salad*
1 cup of cooked asparagus
1 cup of tossed salad
Lo-Cal Salad Dressing
1 pear
No-cal beverage

DINNER
1 cup of Egg Drop Soup*
1½ cups of Asian Stir-Fry*
1 cup of Chinese Fried Rice*
½ cup of pineapple
1 serving of Poppy-Seed Cake*
8 ounces of skim or low-fat milk

MENU 2

BREAKFAST

8 ounces of skim or low-fat milk

1 cup of hot cereal

3 tablespoons of raisins

1 slice of whole-wheat toast

1 tablespoon of peanut butter

Coffee or tea

LUNCH

4 ounces of Pepper Beef Burger*

1 whole-grain bun

1 cup of steamed cauliflower

Spinach Caesar Salad*

1 orange

Coffee or tea

DINNER

6 ounces of Broiled Snapper*

1 small baked potato

1 cup of tossed salad

Lo-Cal Salad Dressing

1 slice of whole-grain bread

1 apple

1 serving of Pineapple Ice*

No-cal beverage

MENU 3

BREAKFAST
8 ounces of skim or low-fat milk
1½ cups of dry cereal
1 banana
1 slice of whole-wheat toast
1 teaspoon of preserves
Coffee or tea

LUNCH
1 cup of soup (your choice)
4 ounces of roast turkey
2 slices of whole-grain bread
Lettuce, sprouts, and Dijon mustard
Unlimited free vegetables
Lo-Cal Salad Dressing
1 pear
No-cal beverage

DINNER
5 ounces of Asian Stir-Fry*
1 cup of steamed carrots
1 slice of whole-grain bread or 1 whole-grain roll
2 Apple-Nut Bran Squares*
8 ounces of skim or low-fat milk
No-cal beverage

MENU 4

BREAKFAST
1 German Fruit Puff*
8 ounces of skim or low-fat milk
Coffee or tea

LUNCH
1 serving of Tuna-Chickpea Salad*
1 cup of broccoli
1 slice of whole-wheat bread
½ cup of brown rice
1 apple
No-cal beverage

DINNER
1 serving of Shrimp and Snow Peas*
1 cup of cooked cabbage
½ cup of Green Beans Almondine
½ cup of sliced apricots
8 ounces of skim or low-fat milk
No-cal beverage

MENU 5

BREAKFAST

8 ounces of skim or low-fat milk

1 cup of berries

1 bagel

2 tablespoons of cream cheese

Coffee or tea

LUNCH

1 cup of Broccoli-Cauliflower Soup*

1 cup of carrots

4 ounces of baked fish

1 slice of whole-grain bread

1 orange

No-cal beverage

DINNER

4 ounces of Slim Southern-Style Fried Chicken*

1 cup of brown rice

1 cup of cooked asparagus

1 cup of tossed salad

Lo-Cal Salad Dressing

2 canned pear halves

No-cal beverage

MENU 6

BREAKFAST

2 Whole-Wheat Breakfast Cakes*
2 tablespoons of maple syrup
8 ounces of skim or low-fat milk
½ grapefruit
Coffee or tea

LUNCH

1 cup of soup (your choice)
2 turkey and sprout sandwiches, open-faced: each
with 1 slice of whole-grain bread, 1 ounce of turkey,
and Dijon mustard
1 cup of brussels sprouts
½ cup of pineapple
1 serving of Pineapple Ice*
No-cal beverage

DINNER

4 ounces of Sesame Scallops*
1 baked potato
Spinach Caesar Salad*
Choice of assorted vegetable relishes: carrots, celery,
radishes, cucumber, etc.
1 slice of Poppy-Seed Cake*
No-cal beverage

I have Learned To Substitute Foods I do Not Like For Foods I do Like in these Recipes. I also made changes For Rachels Diet—
this is a LoT OF FUN and iT changed My Life ~~tomorrow~~

BROCCOLI

¾ pound of fresh chopped broccoli

¾ pound of fresh chopped cauliflower

⅓ cup of chopped onion

1½ cups of bouillon

¼ teaspoon of ground mace

½ teaspoon of salt

⅛ teaspoon of pepper

⅓ cup of shredded Swiss cheese

Cook broccoli, cauliflower, and onion in the bouillon until tender. Pour half the vegetables, along with half the bouillon, into a blender or food processor and blend until smooth. Remove, and blend the remaining vegetable mixture, along with the mace. Return all of blended mixture to pan.

Blend ½ cup of milk with cornstarch and add to vegetables. Add remaining milk, salt, and pepper, and cook until thick and hot, stirring occasionally. Blend in cheese and stir until melted.

Makes 8 servings at 71 calories per serving.

EGG DROP SOUP

1¼ cups of bouillon

1¼ cups of water

2 tablespoons of chopped green onion

1 egg, slightly beaten

Combine bouillon and water in saucepan and bring to boil. Add green onion, and reduce heat. Gently stir in beaten egg, and simmer for 3 minutes or until egg is set. Serve immediately.

Makes 4 servings at 35 calories per serving.

MUSHROOM CLAM CHOWDER

½ cup of fresh mushrooms, chopped

1 teaspoon of vegetable oil

1 7-ounce can of minced clams

½ cup of celery, chopped

⅓ cup of onion, chopped

¼ teaspoon of salt

⅛ teaspoon of pepper

⅛ teaspoon of cayenne

1⅓ cups of nonfat dry milk powder

1½ cups of cold water

1 tablespoon of cornstarch

2 tablespoons of minced fresh parsley

Heat oil in saucepan and sauté mushrooms. Stir in undrained clams, celery, onion, salt, pepper, and cayenne. Cover and let simmer for 5 minutes. Mix together milk powder, water, and cornstarch. (You may substitute 1½ cups of skim milk for the milk powder and water.) Stir milk mixture into saucepan and simmer over low heat until soup thickens. Pour into serving bowls and top each serving with ½ tablespoon of minced parsley.

Makes 4 servings at 142 calories per serving.

VEGETABLE SOUP WITH BARLEY

3	stalks of broccoli (stems only)	1	teaspoon of fenugreek (optional)
1	tablespoon of olive oil	½	teaspoon each of rosemary, thyme, and sage
1	onion, cut in chunks		
2	cloves of garlic, minced		Freshly ground black pepper to taste
2	carrots, cut in chunks		
2	zucchini, cut in chunks	5	cups of low-sodium vegetable bouillon
3	stalks of celery, cut in chunks		
		1	cup of water
8	ounces of sliced mushrooms	⅓	cup of barley, rinsed
1	teaspoon of freshly grated ginger		¼ to ½ teaspoon of salt (optional)
2	bay leaves		

Trim the tough parts from the broccoli stalks and cut in chunks. Save the broccoli florets for another use. In a large pot, sauté the onion and garlic, partially covered, over low heat, for about 3 minutes. Add chopped stalks of broccoli and remaining vegetables to the pot and stir. Add the ginger, bay leaves, and the rest of the spices and stir. Add the bouillon, bring to a boil, then cover and lower heat. Simmer until the vegetables are tender.

Meanwhile, in a small saucepan, bring the 1 cup of water to

a boil, add the barley, lower heat, cover, and cook until barley is done, about 50 minutes. Set this aside. When vegetables are tender, let them cool at least 15 minutes and then purée until smooth. Add the barley to the soup and stir. Add the salt, if desired, and stir. If soup is too thick, add more water. Bring to a boil again and serve.

Makes 10 servings at 67 calories per serving.

Salads

CHICKEN AND SWISS SALAD

½ cup of plain yogurt

2 tablespoons of mayonnaise

1 tablespoon of fresh chopped parsley

1 teaspoon of horseradish

1 teaspoon of prepared mustard

¼ teaspoon of rosemary

¼ teaspoon of garlic powder

1 head of lettuce

12 sliced green pepper rings

6 slices of Swiss cheese, 1 ounce each

6 slices of sweet red onion

6 slices of cooked chicken or turkey, 1 ounce each

24 sliced cucumber rounds, ¼ inch thick

12 tomato slices

Blend together yogurt, mayonnaise, parsley, horseradish, mustard, rosemary, and garlic. Cover and chill while preparing the rest of the salad.

Remove core of lettuce head. Cut lettuce crosswise to get 6 slices, ½ inch thick. Place lettuce slices on serving plates. Top each lettuce slice with 2 green pepper rings, 1 slice of cheese, 1 slice of onion, 1 slice of chicken or turkey, 4 slices of cucumber, and 2 slices of tomato. Top each serving with 2 tablespoons of yogurt mixture.

Makes 6 servings at 224 calories per serving.

POTATO SALAD

3	medium-sized cooked potatoes, diced	1	teaspoon of prepared mustard
¼	cup of chopped green onion	1	teaspoon of dillweed
⅔	cup of chopped celery	½	teaspoon of garlic powder
1	tablespoon of mayonnaise		

Combine all ingredients in a large bowl, and chill at least one hour.

Makes 4 servings, 1 cup each, at 102 calories per serving.

SEASONED TOMATO SALAD

1	cup of fresh chopped tomato	1½	teaspoons of lemon juice
½	teaspoon of basil		Several sprigs of fresh parsley, chopped
½	teaspoon of oregano		

Combine all ingredients, cover, and let marinate in the refrigerator for an hour or more.

Makes 1 serving of 52 calories.

SPINACH CAESAR SALAD

1 clove of garlic

10 ounces of fresh spinach

4 tablespoons of chopped onion

3 tablespoons of mayonnaise

¼ cup of Italian salad dressing

1 tablespoon of lemon or lime juice

¼ teaspoon of salt

⅛ teaspoon of black pepper

3 slices of whole-wheat bread, toasted, cubed

3 tablespoons of grated Parmesan cheese

Cut garlic clove in half and rub salad bowl with the cut ends. Discard garlic. Trim and shred spinach, and add to salad bowl. Add onion. Combine mayonnaise, salad dressing, lemon or lime juice, salt, and pepper, and pour over spinach. Toss warm toasted bread cubes with cheese, and pour onto salad.

Makes 8 servings at 67 calories per serving.

Main Courses

ARTICHOKE-STUFFED PORTOBELLOS

This dish is attractive and tasty enough to serve to guests. It's quick, easy, and low in calories for a main course. While you can use canned artichoke hearts, we like Monterey Farms ArtiHearts, which are vacuum-packed and have both a fresher taste and about half the sodium of canned artichoke hearts.

6 large portobello mushroom caps, whole	6 ounces of artichoke hearts, chopped
6 tablespoons of Newman's Own Olive Oil & Vinegar Dressing	6 tablespoons of shredded cheese (Monterey Jack, cheddar, or Parmesan, for example)
3 tablespoons of Worcestershire sauce	Oregano, black pepper, garlic powder, paprika to taste
2 tablespoons of olive oil, divided	
2 green onions, minced	

Clean the mushroom caps and marinate in the dressing and Worcestershire sauce for at least 2 hours. Preheat oven to 400 degrees. Line shallow baking pan with foil. Drizzle 1 tablespoon of olive oil on foil. Place mushroom caps on foil. Combine all remaining ingredients and spoon evenly into caps. Bake for about 10 to 15 minutes, until mushrooms are tender.

Makes 6 servings at 188 calories per serving.

ASIAN STIR-FRY

¾ pound of top round steak

½ cup of water

2 cups of broccoli florets

2 medium carrots, sliced

1 teaspoon of cornstarch

¼ teaspoon of sugar

2 tablespoons of soy sauce

2 tablespoons of dry sherry

2 tablespoons of cooking oil

1 medium onion, cut into thin wedges

Slice beef across the grain into thin, bite-sized pieces. Set aside. Bring water to a boil, and steam broccoli and carrots over hot water for 3 minutes. In a small bowl or measuring cup, combine cornstarch, sugar, soy sauce, and sherry, and reserve.

Preheat a wok or skillet over high heat for 1 minute. Add 1 tablespoon of the oil. Add vegetables, including onion, and stir-fry for several minutes, until just tender. Remove vegetables. Add remaining oil to skillet. Add beef and brown, stirring constantly. Add soy mixture, still stirring constantly, and stir until sauce thickens. Return vegetables to wok or skillet, cover, and cook 1 minute more.

Makes 4 servings at 292 calories per serving.

BAKED FISH IN SPRING HERBS

1 tablespoon of vegetable oil or butter	1 lemon
1 pound of fish fillets (sole or flounder works best)	1 teaspoon each of dried parsley, chives, and rosemary

Melt butter and pour into shallow baking dish. Arrange fish in dish. Cut lemon in half, and squeeze over the fish about 1 tablespoon of juice from one-half of the lemon. Sprinkle with herbs. Slice the remaining lemon into thin slices, and arrange on top of the fish.

Bake at 500 degrees for 12 to 15 minutes, or until fish flakes easily with fork.

Makes 4 servings of 4 ounces each, at about 115 calories per serving.

BROILED SNAPPER

2 pounds of snapper fillets	1¼ teaspoons of paprika
⅔ cup of tomato juice	⅛ teaspoon of salt
3 tablespoons of vinegar	⅛ teaspoon of black pepper

Cut fillets into 8 pieces. Arrange in shallow baking dish. Combine remaining ingredients and pour over fish. Marinate covered in refrigerator for 1 hour, turning once. Remove fish and place on broiler pan. Brush with marinade and broil 4 to 5 minutes, about

4 inches from heat. Turn and baste again with marinade. Broil another 4 to 5 minutes, or until fish flakes easily with a fork.

Makes 8 servings at 104 calories per serving.

CHICKEN PAPRIKA

1 teaspoon of olive oil

12 ounces of cooked chicken pieces, white meat only (1 pound raw)

1 teaspoon of paprika

⅛ teaspoon of rosemary, crushed

Dash of salt

Dash of black pepper

Garlic powder to taste

Heat oil over medium heat in a small saucepan. Toss in chicken, coating with oil. Stir in seasonings. Serve warm or cold.

Makes 2 to 4 servings: 3 ounces will contain 138 calories, and 6 ounces will contain 276 calories.

CHICKEN SESAME

½ cup of bread crumbs or Pepperidge Farm stuffing mix

⅛ cup of ground sesame seeds

1 clove of garlic, chopped fine

¼ teaspoon each of onion powder, thyme, marjoram, and salt

½ teaspoon of dried parsley

½ teaspoon of dry mustard

⅛ teaspoon of black pepper

3 pounds of chicken pieces, skinned

1 small egg, lightly beaten

Combine dry ingredients and seasonings; mix well. Place a layer of chicken pieces in the bottom of a large casserole dish. Brush the chicken with the beaten egg. Sprinkle with some of the sesame mixture. Continue layering chicken, egg, and sesame mixture until all ingredients are used up.

Bake covered at 300 degrees for 1½ to 2 hours, or until chicken is tender.

Makes 8 servings at approximately 210 calories per serving.

CHICKEN TERIYAKI

1	tablespoon of vegetable oil	1	tablespoon of fresh ginger, grated
2	tablespoons of soy sauce	4	chicken breasts, skinned
1	large clove of garlic, crushed		

Combine all [ingredients in a large bowl] and mix well. Add the chicken and marinate at least 1 hour in the refrigerator, stir[ring occasionally.] Line a baking pan with foil and arrange chicken [pieces on it. Baste each piece with the marinade.] Bake at 350 deg[rees for 45 minutes, or until chicken is tender,] basting frequent[ly with the marinade.]

Makes 4 servi[ngs at 151 calories per serving.]

this is very good

CURRIED LENTILS

This delicious vegetarian dish is well worth the extra time it takes to prepare.

6 tablespoons of olive oil, divided

2 large onions, diced

2 teaspoons of freshly grated ginger

4 or 5 garlic cloves, minced

4 bay leaves

2 teaspoons of ground coriander

2 teaspoons of cumin

1 teaspoon of turmeric

5 cups of water

3 cups of red lentils, rinsed

1 teaspoon of salt

1½ cups of chopped scallions (about 2 bunches)

2 small jalapeño peppers, chopped

6 tablespoons of fresh lime juice

4 tablespoons of chopped fresh cilantro

2 teaspoons of garam masala

In a large saucepan, sauté onions in 2 tablespoons of the olive oil over medium heat, partially covered, for 6 minutes. Add ginger and next 5 ingredients and sauté 1 minute more. Add water and bring to a boil. Then add lentils and salt, bring to a boil again, then lower heat and simmer until lentils are tender and most of the liquid has been absorbed (about 20 minutes). Remove bay leaves, and place the lentils in a large bowl and keep warm. Put remaining 4 tablespoons of olive oil in the saucepan and sauté the scallions and jalapeño peppers over medium heat, partially covered, for 5 minutes. Add to lentil mixture along with the remaining ingredients and combine.

Makes 12 servings at 244 calories per serving.

HALIBUT STEAK WITH VEGETABLES

2 pounds of halibut steaks

Nonstick vegetable cooking spray

⅔ cup of onion, sliced thin

1½ cups of fresh mushrooms, chopped

⅓ cup of tomato, chopped

⅓ cup of green pepper, chopped

¼ cup of fresh parsley, chopped

3 tablespoons of pimiento, chopped

⅓ cup of dry white wine

2 tablespoons of lemon or lime juice

1 teaspoon of salt

¼ teaspoon of dillweed

⅛ teaspoon of pepper

Lemon or lime wedges

Cut steaks into 8 pieces. Spray baking dish with cooking spray. Line bottom of dish with onion. Place fish on top of onion. Combine mushrooms, tomato, green pepper, parsley, and pimiento, and spread over fish. Blend wine, lemon or lime juice, and seasonings, and pour over vegetables. Bake at 350 degrees for 25 minutes, or until fish flakes easily with a fork. Serve with lemon or lime wedges.

Makes 8 servings at 137 calories per serving.

LEAN AND PERFECT PIZZA

Topping

½	pound of extra-lean ground beef	1¼	teaspoons of oregano
1	clove of garlic, minced	1	teaspoon of basil
⅓	cup of chopped onion	½	teaspoon of fennel seed
1	can (16 ounces) of tomatoes, chopped, undrained	⅛	teaspoon of salt
⅓	cup of chopped green pepper	1	cup of shredded mozzarella cheese (4 ounces)

Crust

1	cup of whole-wheat flour	⅓	cup of warm water
½	package of dry yeast	1½	teaspoons of vegetable oil
	Dash of salt		Nonstick vegetable cooking spray

Brown beef, garlic, and onion in saucepan. Drain well. Stir in tomatoes, green pepper, oregano, basil, fennel, and the salt. Bring to a boil. Then reduce heat and simmer gently, uncovered, for 30 minutes.

Meanwhile, combine ⅞ cup of the flour with the yeast and the salt. Add the warm water and oil. Beat at low speed with an electric mixer for 30 seconds, then beat at high speed for 3 minutes. Add as much of the remaining flour as you can stir in with a

spoon. Turn out onto a floured board and knead in enough flour
to make smooth, elastic dough (about 6 minutes). Cover dough
and let stand in a warm place for 10 minutes. Roll dough into a
13-inch circle. Transfer to a pizza pan or a baking sheet sprayed
with cooking spray. Turn up edges of the crust slightly. Bake at
425 degrees for 12 minutes, or until lightly browned.

Pour meat mixture onto crust, top with cheese, and bake for 15
more minutes, or until bubbly. Slice and serve.

Makes 4 servings at 354 calories per serving.

MEDLEY CASSEROLE

2	medium potatoes, cubed (leave skins on!)	½ teaspoon of rosemary
1	medium carrot, sliced in ¼-inch rounds	¼ teaspoon of salt
1	stalk of celery, chopped	¼ teaspoon of black pepper
1	onion, sliced in ¼-inch rounds	1 pound of fish fillets
1½	tablespoons of olive oil	1 medium green pepper, chopped fine
1	teaspoon of dill	1 tablespoon of lemon juice
1	teaspoon of basil	1 medium tomato, chopped fine

Layer potatoes, carrot, celery, and onion in an 8-inch-square
baking dish. Heat oil over medium heat in a small saucepan. Stir
in dill, basil, rosemary, salt, and black pepper. Spoon half of the
seasoned oil over the vegetables. Cover and bake at 425 degrees
for 25 minutes.

Arrange fish fillets on top of the vegetables and sprinkle with lemon juice. Spoon the remaining seasoned oil over the fish. Top with chopped green pepper. Cover and bake for 15 more minutes or until fish flakes easily with a fork. Uncover and add chopped tomato. Bake 5 minutes more, or until tomato is hot and vegetables are tender.

Makes 4 servings at 201 calories per serving.

MRS. DASH COUNTRY CHICKEN AND MUSHROOMS

The list of ingredients in a Mrs. Dash seasoning blend is long. If for some reason you can't find the product in your local grocery, you can substitute a combination of garlic powder, onion powder, black pepper, parsley, basil, oregano, thyme, cayenne pepper, dry mustard, or other herbs and seasonings that you enjoy, to make 3 tablespoons of your own blend.

4 boneless, skinless chicken breasts

1 pound of mushrooms, cleaned, cut in half

2 tablespoons of olive oil

3 tablespoons of Mrs. Dash Garlic & Herb Seasoning Blend

Preheat oven to 375 degrees. Place chicken breasts and mushrooms in two separate bowls. Toss each with 1 tablespoon of olive oil and 1½ tablespoons of Mrs. Dash Garlic & Herb Seasoning Blend. Place each in separate ovenproof casserole dishes and roast 6 to 7 minutes, turning each after 4 minutes. Plate chicken and sprinkle with mushrooms and pan juices.

Makes 4 servings at 225 calories per serving.

MRS. DASH CRUNCHY POPCORN CHICKEN

As mentioned before, the list of ingredients in a Mrs. Dash seasoning blend is long. If for some reason you can't find the product in your local grocery, you can substitute a combination of garlic powder, onion powder, black pepper, sweet chili pepper, chipotle chili pepper, cayenne pepper, cumin, parsley, dry mustard, coriander, and maybe a dash of lime juice and natural smoke flavor, or other herbs and seasonings that you enjoy, to make 3 tablespoons of your own blend.

	Vegetable oil cooking spray		1	cup of dry bread crumbs
2	tablespoons of Mrs. Dash Southwest Chipotle Seasoning Blend		1	egg, lightly beaten
			1	pound of chicken tenders, cut into small pieces

Lightly spray a baking sheet with cooking spray. Preheat oven to 350 degrees. Combine Mrs. Dash Southwest Chipotle Seasoning Blend and bread crumbs in large bowl. Beat egg in another bowl, stir in Mrs. Dash bread-crumb mixture, add chicken, and stir to completely coat chicken. Place chicken pieces on prepared baking sheets, and spray chicken lightly with cooking spray. Bake for 10 minutes, turn and bake a further 10 minutes, remove, and serve warm.

Makes 4 servings at 250 calories per serving.

PAPRIKA PORK GOULASH

1	pound of pork tenderloin	1	tablespoon of cornstarch
	Nonstick vegetable cooking spray	1	cup of plain yogurt
		¼	cup of fresh parsley
1	large onion, chopped	2½	cups of cooked whole-wheat noodles
¾	cup of bouillon		
1	tablespoon of paprika		

Trim all visible fat from pork. Slice pork diagonally into ¼-inch slices. Spray skillet with cooking spray, and heat over medium heat. Brown meat in skillet, stirring occasionally. Remove meat from pan. Place onions in pan and cook lightly until clear. (You may add some of the bouillon if there isn't enough fat to cook the onions.)

Return meat to skillet. Add bouillon and paprika. Cover and let simmer 15 to 20 minutes, until pork is tender. Take 6 table-spoons of bouillon out of pan and reserve in small container in refrigerator.

Blend cornstarch into yogurt in a small bowl. Take the reserved bouillon out of the refrigerator and stir into the yogurt mixture, 1 tablespoon at a time. Add yogurt mixture to skillet and heat through. Stir in parsley, and serve over hot noodles.

Makes 5 servings at 296 calories per serving.

PEPPER BEEF BURGERS

¼	cup of fine dry bread crumbs	¾	pound of ground chuck or ground round
2	tablespoons of low-fat dry milk	2	medium onions, sliced thin
½	teaspoon of basil	¾	cup of tomato sauce
½	teaspoon of oregano	¼	cup of red wine
½	teaspoon of garlic powder	1	large green pepper, julienned
⅛	teaspoon of salt		
⅛	teaspoon of black pepper		

Combine bread crumbs, milk, and seasonings in bowl. Add meat and mix well. Shape into four patties, ¾ inch thick. Brown patties on both sides in skillet. Drain off fat. Add onions to skillet. Blend together tomato sauce and wine, and pour into skillet. Cover and cook on low heat for about 10 minutes. Top with green pepper, cover, and cook 10 minutes more.

Makes 4 servings at 219 calories per serving.

QUICK SKILLET

2   cups of lean roasted pork, cut into 1-inch cubes

2   onions, cut into chunks

2   tablespoons of soy sauce

2   tablespoons of water

¼   cup of unsweetened pineapple juice

¾   pound of fresh asparagus, cut into 1-inch lengths

⅓   cup of fresh mushrooms, sliced

¾   cup of cubed tomato pieces

1   teaspoon of cornstarch

¼   cup of white wine or vinegar

Combine pork, onions, soy sauce, and water in skillet. Cook on high heat for 1 or 2 minutes. Add juice, asparagus, and mushrooms, and cook 6 minutes more. Add tomato. Dissolve cornstarch in wine and stir into meat mixture. Stirring constantly, cook for 2 or 3 minutes more, until sauce thickens, and vegetables are tender.

Makes 4 servings at 257 calories per serving.

SALMON LOAF

1 tablespoon of olive oil, plus 1 teaspoon, separated

2 cans (7½ ounces each) of no-salt-added salmon, with juice

2 scallions, chopped

1 clove of garlic, minced

1 large stalk of celery, chopped fine

½ red bell pepper, chopped fine

½ cup of oats

¾ cup of Pepperidge Farm stuffing mix, or bread crumbs

1 tablespoon of lemon juice

½ cup of Egg Beaters

1 tablespoon of steak sauce

1 tablespoon of dried parsley flakes

2 tablespoon of Mrs. Dash chicken seasoning

1 teaspoon of dry mustard powder

Freshly ground black pepper to taste

Paprika

Preheat oven to 350 degrees. With the 1 teaspoon of olive oil, lightly oil a loaf pan or similar casserole. In a large bowl, combine all other ingredients except paprika. Put in oiled loaf pan or casserole and sprinkle with paprika. Before baking, use a spatula, flipper, or other tool to press loaf slightly away from the sides of the pan. Bake about 45 minutes or until a crust forms. Let rest for 20 minutes. Then cut around the edges to loosen from pan and invert onto a serving plate.

Makes 8 servings at 142 calories per serving.

SALMON WITH DILL

This dish is also good cold.

2 tablespoons of olive oil

1 tablespoon of dill

2 teaspoons of garlic powder

Black pepper to taste

1 tablespoon of lemon juice

1½ pounds of salmon fillets

Line baking pan with foil. Drizzle olive oil onto foil. Sprinkle with seasonings and lemon juice. Add fish and swish both sides of each piece around in the seasonings and oil. Bake at 400 degrees for about 15 minutes, until fish flakes easily with a fork.

Makes 4 servings at 311 calories per serving, or 6 servings at 208 calories per serving.

SEAFOOD ITALIA

Nonstick vegetable cooking spray

2 pounds of fish fillets

¼ cup of unsalted tomato juice

3 tablespoons of steak sauce

1½ tablespoons of Italian salad dressing

⅛ teaspoon of curry powder

Dash of hot pepper sauce

Spray nonstick broiler pan with cooking spray. Arrange fillets on pan. Combine remaining ingredients, and pour half of mixture over the fish. Broil 4 to 5 minutes, then turn fillets over, cover with the remaining sauce, and broil another 4 to 5 minutes, or until fish flakes easily with a fork.

Makes 8 servings of 4 ounces each, including sauce, at 109 calories per serving.

SESAME SCALLOPS

3	tablespoons of sherry	
2	tablespoons of cooking oil	
1	tablespoon of sesame seeds, crushed	
2	teaspoons of grated onion	
1	clove of garlic, crushed	
¼	teaspoon of salt	
⅛	teaspoon of black pepper	

1   pound of large fresh scallops

1   green pepper, cut into chunks

1   sweet red pepper, cut into chunks

1   can (8 ounces) of unsweetened pineapple chunks, drained

12   cherry tomatoes

Combine sherry, oil, sesame seeds, onion, garlic, salt, and black pepper in large plastic bowl. Add scallops and pepper chunks, and marinate in refrigerator for 3 or 4 hours, stirring occasionally. Thread scallops, peppers, and pineapple on 6 skewers. Place skewers in baking pan and pour marinade in. Bake at 425 degrees for 10 minutes, or until scallops are tender, turning skewers occasionally. Place two tomatoes on the end of each skewer, and return to oven for 5 more minutes.

Makes 6 servings at about 174 calories per serving.

SHRIMP AND SNOW PEAS

To enjoy Asian-style cooking while cutting back on sodium, try Bragg Liquid Aminos, available at health food stores. It's made from soy but has less sodium than even low-sodium soy sauces.

1 tablespoon of olive oil

1 small yellow onion, chopped

4 green onions, chopped

1 ½-inch piece of fresh ginger, minced (about 1 teaspoon)

4 cloves of garlic, minced

1 teaspoon of minced jalapeño pepper

1 carrot, julienned

½ cup of snow peas

A few tablespoons of water

6 ounces of sliced mushrooms

1 pound of shrimp, shelled and deveined

A dash of sesame oil

1 tablespoon of Bragg Liquid Aminos

Black pepper to taste

3 cups of cooked rice

Heat the olive oil in a large skillet over medium heat, then add the yellow onion and cook, stirring often, until translucent. Add the remaining vegetables and spices one at a time, heating for about a minute before adding the next. Add the water with the mushrooms, stir, reduce heat, and let cook for a few minutes, until mushrooms are tender. Add shrimp and cook, stirring often, until it is pink and tightly curled and the vegetables are tender. Add sesame oil, Liquid Aminos, and black pepper and stir. Serve over ½ cup of rice per serving.

Makes 6 servings at 300 calories per serving.

SHRIMP JAMBALAYA

2 tablespoons of olive oil

½ cup of chopped green onion

¼ cup of chopped green pepper

1 clove of garlic, minced

2 tablespoons of whole-wheat flour

1 can (16 ounces) of stewed tomatoes, undrained

1 cup of cooked, cubed ham

½ cup of water

2 bay leaves

½ teaspoon of thyme

½ teaspoon of basil

¼ teaspoon of dillweed

¼ teaspoon of crushed red pepper

¼ teaspoon of salt

⅛ teaspoon of black pepper

Dash of Tobasco sauce

1 cup of uncooked brown rice, washed and drained

1 pound of shelled shrimp

Heat oil in saucepan and brown onion, green pepper, and garlic until tender. Blend in all remaining ingredients except the shrimp. Bring to a boil, then reduce heat and simmer for about 30 minutes, stirring frequently. Add shrimp and cook 15 minutes more, or until rice and shrimp are cooked.

Makes 6 servings at 283 calories per serving.

SLIM SOUTHERN-STYLE FRIED CHICKEN

4   pounds of chicken
    pieces, skinned
    Water
½   cup of bread crumbs
½   teaspoon of paprika
¼   teaspoon of salt

¼   teaspoon of thyme
¼   teaspoon of marjoram
¼   teaspoon of celery seed
⅛   teaspoon of black
    pepper

Brush chicken pieces with water to moisten. Combine remaining ingredients in a large bowl. Dredge chicken in the coating, and arrange on a nonstick baking sheet. Bake at 375 degrees for 45 minutes, or until crisp on the outside and tender inside.

Makes 8 servings at about 186 calories per serving.

SPICY ORANGE PORK

6   pork chops, top loin,
    ½ inch thick
    Nonstick vegetable
    spray
¼   teaspoon of salt
¼   teaspoon of pepper
1¼ cup of unsweetened
    orange juice

2   medium oranges
1   cup of water
2   teaspoons of sugar
1   tablespoon of
    cornstarch
¼   teaspoon of allspice

Trim pork chops of all visible fat. Spray skillet with nonstick vegetable spray, and heat over medium heat. Brown chops on both sides. Sprinkle with salt and pepper, and add ¼ cup of the orange juice. Cover and let simmer 25 minutes or until tender.

Meanwhile, remove a thin layer of peel from one orange, and julienne the peel. Simmer strips in water for 15 minutes, drain, and set aside. Peel and section both oranges, and cut the sections into ½-inch chunks.

Combine sugar, cornstarch, and the remaining 1 cup of orange juice in another saucepan, stirring constantly over medium heat until thickened. Add the julienned orange peel, orange chunks, and allspice. Simmer 1 or 2 minutes longer, stirring occasionally. Remove chops to serving dish, and top with sauce.

Makes 6 servings at 205 calories per serving.

TUNA-CHICKPEA SALAD

This main dish is equally delicious when made with canned salmon. I use no-salt-added tuna, chickpeas, and prepared mustard.

1	can (15 ounces) of chickpeas, drained	¼	cup of Newman's Own Olive Oil & Vinegar Dressing
2	cans (6 ounces each) of water-packed tuna, drained	4	scallions, chopped
2	cloves of garlic	2	stalks of celery, thinly sliced
1	teaspoon of freshly grated ginger	¼	cup of chopped fresh parsley
1	tablespoon of fresh lemon juice		Grated rind of ½ lemon
1	teaspoon of dried dill	¼	teaspoon of salt (optional)
½	teaspoon of dried thyme		Freshly ground black pepper to taste
1	tablespoon of prepared no-salt mustard		

In a food processor, process the chickpeas, tuna, garlic, ginger, lemon juice, dill, thyme, mustard, and the olive oil and vinegar dressing until fairly smooth. Add all other ingredients and mix well. Chill about one hour before serving. Makes 4 servings at 238 calories per serving or 6 servings at 159 calories per serving.

Vegetables

CHINESE FRIED RICE

2	cups of water	¼	cup of water
1	cup of brown rice	¾	cup of celery, chopped
	Nonstick vegetable cooking spray	½	cup of green pepper, chopped
2	eggs, beaten	1	clove of garlic, minced
2	large onions, chopped	3	green onions, chopped
2	teaspoons of vegetable oil		

Bring 2 cups of water to a boil, add rice, and reduce heat. Let simmer for 40 to 45 minutes, until tender. Set aside.

Spray a large skillet with cooking spray. Add eggs and cook over low heat without stirring. When eggs are set, remove from skillet, crumble with a fork, and reserve. Brown onions in skillet with the oil. Add remaining ingredients, and heat to boiling. Add cooked rice. Reduce heat and simmer 1 minute. Stir in egg. Remove from heat, cover, and let stand 5 minutes.

Makes 8 servings at 92 calories per serving.

CITRUS CARROTS

1 cup of carrots	2 teaspoons of fresh lemon juice
¼ cup of water	
1 tablespoon of fresh orange juice	2 lemon slices
	4 orange slices

Cut carrots in quarters lengthwise, then cut into 1-inch strips. Bring water to a boil in saucepan. Place carrots in water, reduce heat, cover, and cook until just tender. Add juices and stir. Place sliced lemon and orange rounds on top of carrots, cover, and cook 2 or 3 minutes more.

Makes one serving of 52 calories.

OVEN-FRIED POTATOES

4 medium potatoes, skins on	⅛ teaspoon of onion powder
1 tablespoon of oil	1 to 1½ teaspoons of paprika (to taste)
⅛ teaspoon of garlic powder	Salt and pepper to taste

Slice potatoes lengthwise into eighths.

Line a shallow baking pan with foil, and put all ingredients into the pan, tossing well to coat the potatoes with the oil and seasonings.

Bake at 325 degrees for 1 hour, or at a higher temperature for less time if you wish. Adjust seasonings if necessary.

Makes 4 servings at 115 calories per serving.

POLENTA

Polenta can be served as a hot breakfast cereal as well as a side dish for lunch or dinner. Once cool, polenta can be sliced and reheated. Some polenta recipes use less liquid, but the 4 cups used here make a creamier dish. Owing to its mild flavor, you can use just about any seasoning or sauce to dress it up. Here I offer a basic polenta recipe, followed by a variation that uses one of my favorite seasoning combinations.

Basic Polenta

4 cups of bouillon	1 tablespoon of olive oil
1 cup of dry polenta or cornmeal	¼ teaspoon of salt

In medium-sized pot, bring bouillon to boil. Gradually stir in the polenta. Reduce heat, add the oil and salt, and let simmer, stirring often, for 15 to 20 minutes. Serve immediately or pour into a lightly oiled loaf pan, or shallow baking pan if you prefer, and let cool. Refrigerate until ready to slice and reheat.

Seasoned Polenta

Make Basic Polenta, adding the following seasonings along with the oil and salt:

1½ teaspoons of dried minced garlic (or substitute a couple of fresh cloves, minced)

1 teaspoon of dried minced onion powder

½ teaspoon of crushed dried red pepper

¼ teaspoon of dried lemon peel

½ teaspoon of dried basil

½ teaspoon of dried oregano

½ teaspoon of paprika

¼ teaspoon of dried thyme

A dash of ground ginger

Freshly ground black pepper to taste

Makes 8 servings at 88 calories per serving.

SPICY GREEN BEANS

¾ pound of fresh whole green beans

¾ cup of unsalted tomato juice

2 tablespoons of chopped onion

1 teaspoon of oregano

½ teaspoon of basil

¼ teaspoon of garlic powder

¼ teaspoon of salt

⅛ teaspoon of pepper

1 tablespoon of grated Romano cheese

Wash and trim green beans and cut into 1-inch lengths. Combine beans and remaining ingredients in saucepan and bring to a boil. Reduce heat and simmer, covered, for 5 minutes. Uncover and continue to cook until beans are tender. Sprinkle with cheese.

Makes 3 servings at 47 calories per serving.

STOVETOP SPINACH CASSEROLE

¾ pound of fresh spinach

½ cup of chicken or vegetable bouillon

2 tablespoons of mayonnaise

3 tablespoons of fresh onion, chopped fine

Wash and trim spinach. Combine all ingredients in saucepan, and bring to a boil. Reduce heat immediately and simmer, uncovered, until most of the liquid has evaporated.

Makes 3 servings at 44 calories per serving.

SUCCOTASH

The beans and corn make this a great vegetarian main or side dish. Serving suggestion: top with grated cheddar cheese (add 28 calories per tablespoon).

1   medium onion, chopped

1   tablespoon of olive oil

4   cloves of garlic, minced

1   red bell pepper, chopped

1   yellow bell pepper, chopped

1   bunch of fresh asparagus, chopped

15 ounces of canned or frozen no-salt-added lima, butter, garbanzo, or cannellini beans

15 ounces of canned or frozen no-salt-added corn

1   teaspoon of dried thyme

1   teaspoon of paprika

Dash of cayenne

Freshly ground black pepper to taste

2   tablespoons of fresh parsley, chopped

Sauté onion in oil over medium heat, stirring often, until onion is translucent. Add garlic and cook 1 minute more. Add bell peppers and asparagus. Cook for about 10 minutes, stirring occasionally. Drain beans and corn and add to skillet. (If using frozen beans and corn, simply add them to the skillet, and they will thaw quickly.) Heat through. Add seasonings and serve.

Makes 8 main-dish servings at 115 calories per serving or 12 side-dish servings at 77 calories per serving.

Desserts

APPLE-NUT BRAN SQUARES

1   cup of 40% Bran
     Flakes or Raisin Bran

½   cup of wheat germ

½   cup of nonfat dry milk
     powder

½   teaspoon of baking
     powder

⅛   teaspoon of salt

2   beaten eggs

½   cup of firmly packed
     brown sugar

½   cup of finely chopped
     apples, skins on

2   tablespoons of
     vegetable oil

1   tablespoon of dark
     molasses

1¾   teaspoons of vanilla

⅓   cup of chopped pecans
     or walnuts

     Nonstick vegetable
     cooking spray

Combine bran, wheat germ, milk, baking powder, and salt in a large bowl. In a separate bowl, combine eggs, sugar, apples, oil, molasses, and vanilla. Add egg mixture gradually to dry mixture, blending well. Add nuts. Spray a 9-inch-square baking pan with cooking spray. Turn batter into pan and bake at 350 degrees for 25 minutes. Cool and cut into 20 squares.

Makes 20 servings at approximately 85 calories per serving.

BREAD PUDDING

1	teaspoon of olive oil	½	teaspoon of nutmeg
6	cups of whole-wheat bread, cubed	1	teaspoon of cinnamon
3	cups of skim milk	1	apple, diced
¾	cup of Egg Beaters	¼	cup of raisins
½	cup of brown sugar, packed	1	tablespoon of lemon juice
½	teaspoon of ginger	1	teaspoon of vanilla

Preheat oven to 325 degrees. Use the olive oil to coat a 9- by 11- by 2-inch baking dish. Place the bread and milk in a large mixing bowl. Let soak for 15 minutes. In another bowl, mix all other ingredients. Pour over soaked bread and stir lightly to combine. Pour into baking dish and bake for 45 to 60 minutes until set. Serve warm or cold.

Makes 12 servings at 145 calories per serving.

PINEAPPLE ICE

This recipe is also refreshing when frozen into ice-cube trays and served in beverages.

1	large, ripe pineapple, cut into chunks	2 to 4 tablespoons of honey (optional)
2	teaspoons of lemon juice	

Place the pineapple chunks and lemon juice (and honey if the fruit is not very sweet) in a blender or food processor. Purée until smooth. Pour into a plastic freezer container or ice-cube trays and freeze for about 1 hour. When mixture is slushy-frozen, purée again in blender until creamy. Pour back into freezer container or ice-cube trays and freeze at least 2 hours more.

Makes 6 to 8 servings depending on the size of the pineapple, at 54 calories per ½-cup serving.

POPPY-SEED CAKE

	Nonstick vegetable cooking spray	1	cup of whole-wheat flour
	Small amount of whole-wheat flour	½	teaspoon of salt
⅓	cup of vegetable oil	½	teaspoon of baking soda
¾	cup of granulated white sugar	⅔	cup of plain low-fat yogurt
2	eggs, separated	⅓	cup of poppy seeds
1	teaspoon of vanilla		

Spray an 8-inch tube pan with nonstick vegetable cooking spray, and dust lightly with whole-wheat flour. Blend the oil and sugar in a large bowl. Add the egg yolks one at a time, beating well after each addition. Add the vanilla. In another bowl, sift together the flour, salt, and baking soda. Alternately fold the flour mixture and the yogurt into the oil and sugar mixture. Set aside. Beat the egg whites until stiff. Fold into the batter. Fold in the poppy seeds. Pour the batter into the pan. Bake at 350 degrees for about 45 minutes, until the top is nicely brown and a tooth-pick inserted in the center comes out clean.

Makes 20 servings at 106 calories per ⅜-inch-thick slice.

Crackers and Pancakes

GERMAN FRUIT PUFF

½ cup of all-purpose flour

½ cup of whole-wheat flour

½ teaspoon of baking powder

½ teaspoon of salt

1 cup of skim milk

5 eggs

2 teaspoons of vegetable oil

3¼ cups of any variety of fresh fruit, sliced

Preheat oven to 425 degrees. Sift together flours, baking powder, and salt in mixing bowl. Stir in milk. Beat eggs in, one at a time. Heat oil over medium heat in a large, metal-handled skillet. Pour in batter and let cook 1 minute. Place skillet in oven and bake, uncovered, for 20 minutes, or until puff is golden brown. Top with fruit, and slice into 6 wedges.

Makes 6 servings at 207 calories per serving.

TOASTED OAT THINS

½ cup of quick-cooking rolled oats

⅓ cup of all-purpose unbleached, enriched flour

⅓ cup of whole-wheat flour

⅓ cup of wheat germ

1 tablespoon of sugar

1 tablespoon of sesame seeds, crushed

½ teaspoon of garlic powder

⅛ teaspoon of salt

¼ cup of butter

½ cup of cold water

Blend oats in a blender or food processor until evenly ground. Pour oats into mixing bowl. Add flours, wheat germ, sugar, sesame seed, garlic, and salt. Cut in butter until mixture has consistency of coarse bread crumbs. Gradually mix in cold water to form a dough. Shape the dough into a 9-inch-long roll. Wrap in plastic wrap and chill for at least 3 hours. Slice into ⅛-inch-thick rounds and place on foil-lined, ungreased baking sheet. Flatten with tines of a fork until thin. Bake at 375 degrees for 12 minutes, or until edges are nicely browned. Cool on wire rack.

Makes 6-dozen crackers at 19 calories each.

WHOLE-WHEAT BREAKFAST CAKES

1¼	cups of whole-wheat flour	1	egg
2¼	teaspoons of baking powder	1¼	cups of skim milk
¼	teaspoon of salt		Nonstick vegetable cooking spray

Combine flour, baking powder, and salt in mixing bowl. Beat together egg and milk, and stir into flour mixture to form lumpy batter. Spray nonstick skillet with cooking spray and heat over medium heat. Drop batter by spoonfuls onto skillet to make 4-inch pancakes. Reduce heat to low and cook until bubbles begin to form on cakes. Turn and cook on the other side until golden brown.

Makes 8 servings of cake at about 87 calories each.

12

EPILOGUE

I have focused a great deal of effort in this updated edition to help overweight people who have lost weight on the Rotation Diet avoid a rebound weight gain and meet the lifetime challenge of weight maintenance. I want to especially recommend the websites of two nonprofit organizations that can give you ongoing help in your efforts:

- America on the Move: www.americaonthemove.org. This website offers tips on healthy eating and simple ways to increase the number of steps you take. You can sign up for free, buy a step counter, and find out about local organizational activities in your area.
- National Weight Control Registry: www.nwcr.ws. When you have lost 30 pounds and kept the weight off for a year, you can become a member of the registry. Membership can help you maintain your weight loss.

You will find much additional information about organizations and other websites that can offer continuing help in preventing weight gain in the Resources section of this book.

Good luck.

Acknowledgments

I am greatly indebted to my many colleagues and students who contributed so much to the work we did in helping overweight people when I was director of the Weight Management Program at Vanderbilt. Without their help, the Rotation Diet would never have been created.

To begin with, it was my former student Dr. Gordon Kaplan who used the term *weight management* when he recruited participants for his dissertation study on the factors that lead to long-term success in weight management. This study led to the creation of the Weight Management Program. Dr. Kenneth Wallston soon joined us and assumed primary responsibility for the overall design of the program's research. Dr. David Schlundt contributed an analysis of eating and activity problem areas, and I have adapted many of his ideas in Chapter 10. Dr. Craig Heim, then director of the Center for Health Promotion at Vanderbilt Medical School, supervised the medical research on the health benefits of the Rotation Diet that are reported in Chapter 1.

Another former student, Dr. Mark McMinn, contributed greatly with his studies of the biochemical factors that underlie the problem of obesity. Three of my former graduate students, Ruth Daby, Tracy Sbrocco, and Crystal Sulyma, assisted in the leadership of weight-management groups and contributed to some of the material in Chapter 10.

The nutrition consultant to the program, Rachel Willis, RD, helped in the design of the original Alternate Menus for the Rotation Diet in Chapter 11. Joyce Weingartner created the unique bread recipes in Chapter 7.

Thanks to Summer Davis for her years as administrator and office manager of the program. Her personal experience and understanding of the special problems that women face in managing their weight, and her knowledge of how those problems are intertwined with other aspects of their lives, enriched us all and contributed to our ability as leaders.

Two experts in the obesity field have been especially helpful to me in this update to *The Rotation Diet*. Jamie Pope, MS, RD, lecturer in the Vanderbilt School of Nursing, has kept me advised on the latest research on diet and obesity. Dr. Maiej Buchowski, research professor of medicine and pediatrics and director of the Energy Balance Laboratory at Vanderbilt Medical School, has been kind enough to read and critique the draft chapters on physical activity and metabolism. Any errors that remain in these chapters are my responsibility.

I don't know what I did to deserve them, but I have a very special family. Words can do little to express my love and appreciation for their being so supportive when I lost 75 pounds forty-eight years ago and for helping me maintain an environment that keeps it all off. For this new edition of *The Rotation Diet* I want to thank my wife, Enid, and daughter, Reyna Lorele, for the care they have taken in creating and testing many delicious new recipes. Reyna also helped integrate the comments and suggestions of my editor into the manuscript.

W. W. Norton has published all of my books since we first made contact thirty years ago. I had the critical editorial advice of Starling Lawrence for the first edition of this book. Amy Cherry took over for this revision and update. Both had the challenging task of untwisting my convoluted style and making some complex information more comprehensible. In addition to Amy Cherry, I want to thank Laura Romain, Nancy Palmquist, Susan Sanfrey, Louise Mattarelliano, and Sue Carlson for their collaboration in the book's production.

I want to express my deep appreciation to Richard Pine once again for his help in my thirty years of writing and publishing. After I had contacted six publishers with my first book, *The 200 Calorie Solution*, and been turned down because they felt it lacked "commercial" value, Richard and his father, Arthur, took me under their wing. They introduced me to Starling Lawrence, who read the manuscript and thought I had something worthwhile to say. The support I have received from Richard and the editors at W. W. Norton is truly appreciated. I have updated and incorporated some important information from *The 200 Calorie Solution* into this new edition of *The Rotation Diet*.

Finally, I want to thank the folks at ESHA Research for the help they have given me in the twenty-three years I have been using *the Food Processor nutrition and fitness software.* The latest instance occurred when gremlins attacked my computer and paralyzed the program late one afternoon as I began work on this update. It took but one phone call, and Patrick Murphy from tech support had me up and running again the next morning.

Appendix A

CALORIE, FAT GRAM, AND FIBER COUNTER

HOW TO USE THE COUNTER

Food items are in alphabetical order within a number of different food categories. The categories are as follows, with the page numbers on which you will find them.

Beverages   306
Breads and Flours   307–10
Candy   310–12
Cereals   312–14
Cheeses   314–15
Combination Foods   315–20
Desserts and Toppings   320–24
Eggs   325
Fast Food   325–27
Fats   327–28
Fish   328–32
Fruit   332–34
Fruit Juices and Nectars   334–35

Gravies, Sauces, and Dips   335–37

Meats   337–41

Milk and Yogurt   342–43

Miscellaneous   343–44

Nuts and Seeds   344

Pasta and Rice   344–45

Poultry   345–46

Salad Dressings   346–47

Snack Foods   347–48

Soups   348–51

Vegetables   351–55

Vegetable Salads   355–56

Foods are listed in the portion sizes commonly consumed. Information is given for the total amount of fat in grams, total number of calories, and number of grams of fiber. I have included a wide sampling of generic foods and beverages. If you cannot find a product in this counter or you use a specific brand, consult the nutrition labeling that appears on the food product. The extensive list of combination foods in this appendix represents items from different food manufacturers, or an average from several, without naming them (for example, lasagna or macaroni and cheese). Combination foods may be listed as "hmde" (homemade) or "frzn" (frozen). Values for these dishes, soups, salads, and sandwiches represent the ingredients from traditional recipes. For most "lighter" versions, nutrition counts can be found with the recipe in cookbooks or magazines. If you create your own lower-fat recipes, simply add up the nutrition counts for the ingredients and then divide by the number of servings the recipe yields.

Note on Fast Foods: Fast-food restaurants frequently change their menus and the nutritional values of similarly named foods. For comprehensive, up-to-date listings of nutritional information for items offered by the major fast-food restaurants, check their websites. Books such as Corrine T. Netzer's *The Complete Book of Food Counts* list many fast-food items.

Item	Serving	Total Fat (g)	Calories	Fiber (g)
Beverages				
beer				
regular*	12 fl. oz.	0	148	0
light*	12 fl. oz.	0	100	0
nonalcoholic	12 fl. oz.	0	90	0
carbonated drink				
regular	12 fl. oz.	0	152	0
sugar free	12 fl. oz.	0	1	0
club soda/seltzer	12 fl. oz.	0	0	0
coffee, brewed or instant	8 fl. oz.	0	4	0
eggnog, nonalcoholic				
w/ whole milk	8 fl. oz.	19.0	342	0
w/ 2% milk	8 fl. oz.	8.1	188	0
fruit punch	8 fl. oz.	0	107	0
gin, 90 proof*	1 fl. oz.	0	70	0
grape juice drink, canned	6 fl. oz.	0	89	0
Kool-Aid, from mix, any flavor	8 fl. oz.	0	95	0
lemonade, mix or frzn	8 fl. oz.	0	102	0
lemonade, sugar free	8 fl. oz.	0	4	0
rum, 80 proof*	1 fl. oz.	0	70	0
tea, brewed or instant	8 fl. oz.	0	0	0
tonic water	8 fl. oz.	0	90	0
vodka, 80 proof*	1 fl. oz.	0	70	0
whiskey, 86 proof*	1 fl. oz.	0	70	0
wine*				
dessert and apertif	4 fl. oz.	0	184	0
red or rosé	4 fl. oz.	0	85	0
white, dry or medium	4 fl. oz.	0	80	0
wine cooler	8 fl. oz.	0	83	0

* Although alcohol contains no fat, scientific evidence suggests that it may facilitate fat storage and hamper your weight-loss efforts. Excessive alcohol intake is detrimental to your health. We concur with other health organizations in recommending discretion in the use of alcoholic beverages.

Item	Serving	Total Fat (g)	Calories	Fiber (g)
Breads and Flours				
bagel, cinnamon raisin	1 medium	1.2	195	2
bagel, plain	1 medium	1.1	180	2
barley flour	1 cup	3.0	600	31
biscuit				
baking powder	1 medium	6.6	156	1
buttermilk	1 medium	5.8	127	1
bread				
French/Vienna	1 slice	1.0	90	1
fruit w/ nuts	1 slice	10.1	210	1
fruit w/o nuts	1 slice	5.9	150	1
Italian	1 slice	0.5	80	1
mixed grain	1 slice	0.9	70	2
multigrain, "lite"	1 slice	0.5	45	3
pita, plain	1 large	0.7	165	2
pita, whole wheat	1 large	1.2	180	7
raisin	1 slice	1.1	70	1
rye, American	1 slice	0.9	66	2
rye, pumpernickel	1 slice	0.8	82	2
sourdough	1 slice	0.8	70	1
wheat, commercial	1 slice	1.1	75	2
wheat, "lite"	1 slice	0.5	45	3
white, commercial	1 slice	1.0	75	0
white, hmde	1 slice	1.7	72	0
white, "lite"	1 slice	0.5	42	2
whole wheat, commercial	1 slice	1.2	80	3
bread crumbs	1 cup	5.4	395	4
breadsticks				
plain	1 small	0.3	39	0
sesame	1 small	2.2	51	0
bulgur, dry	1 cup	2.0	477	25
coffee cake	1 piece	7.0	233	1
cornbread				
from mix	⅛ mix	4.0	160	1
hmde	1 piece	7.3	198	2
cornflake crumbs	1 oz.	0	100	1
crackers				
Captain's Wafers	4 crackers	2.0	60	0
cheese	5 pieces	4.9	81	0
Cheese Nips	13 crackers	3.2	70	0

Item	Serving	Total Fat (g)	Calories	Fiber (g)
cheese w/ peanut butter	2 oz. pkg.	13.5	283	1
Goldfish, any flavor	12 crackers	2.0	34	0
graham	2 squares	1.3	60	0
graham, crumbs	½ cup	6.1	250	2
matzohs	1 board	0.4	112	0
melba toast	1 piece	0.2	20	0
Norwegian flatbread	2 thin	0.2	40	0
oyster	33 crackers	3.8	143	0
rice cakes	1 piece	0.2	35	0
rice wafer	3 wafers	0	31	0
Ritz	3 crackers	3.0	53	0
RyKrisp, plain	2 crackers	0.2	40	2
saltines	2 crackers	0.7	26	0
sesame wafers	3 crackers	3.0	70	0
soda	5 crackers	1.9	63	0
toasted w/ peanut butter	1.5 oz. pkg.	10.5	212	0
Triscuit	2 crackers	1.6	40	1
Wasa crispbread	1 piece	1.0	45	1
Wheat Thins	4 crackers	1.5	35	0
wheat w/ cheese	1.5 oz. pkg.	10.9	212	0
Wheatsworth	5 crackers	3.0	70	1
zwieback	2 crackers	1.2	60	0
crepe	1 medium	12.5	230	0
croissant	1 medium	11.5	167	1
croutons, commercial	¼ cup	1.8	50	1
Danish pastry	1 medium	19.3	256	1
doughnut				
cake	1 2.2 oz.	16.2	250	1
yeast	1 2.2 oz.	13.3	235	1
dumpling, plain	1 medium	1.1	42	0
English muffin				
plain	1	1.1	135	1
w/ raisins	1	1.2	150	1
whole wheat	1	2.0	170	2
flour				
rye, medium	1 cup	2.2	400	13
soy	1 cup	18.0	380	2
white, all purpose	1 cup	1.2	455	4
white, bread	1 cup	3.0	401	4
white, self-rising	1 cup	1.2	436	4
whole wheat	1 cup	2.3	400	14

Item	Serving	Total Fat (g)	Calories	Fiber (g)
French toast				
frzn variety	1 slice	6.0	139	0
hmde	1 slice	10.7	172	1
funnel cake	6 in. diam.	15.3	285	1
hush puppy	1 medium	5.5	153	1
matzoh ball	1	7.6	121	0
muffins				
all types, commercial	1 large (3 oz.)	10.3	242	1
banana nut	1 medium	5.0	135	2
blueberry, from mix	1 medium	5.1	131	1
bran, hmde	1 medium	5.8	130	3
corn	1 medium	4.8	175	2
white, plain	1 medium	5.4	135	1
pancakes				
buckwheat, from mix	3 medium	12.3	270	3
buttermilk, from mix	3 medium	10.0	270	2
hmde	3 medium	9.6	312	2
"lite," from mix	3 medium	2.0	190	5
whole wheat, from mix	3 medium	3.0	180	6
phyllo dough	2 oz.	3.4	170	1
pie crust, plain	⅛ pie	8.0	125	0
popover	1	5.0	170	0
rice bran	1 oz.	0.4	80	2
rolls				
brown & serve	1	2.2	100	0
cloverleaf	1	3.2	89	0
crescent	1	5.6	102	1
croissant	1 small	6.0	120	0
French	1	0.4	137	1
hamburger	1	3.0	180	1
hard	1	1.2	115	1
hot dog	1	2.1	116	1
kaiser/hoagie	1 medium	2.0	190	1
pan type	1 small	1.0	80	0
parkerhouse	1	2.1	59	0
raisin	1 large	1.9	179	1
rye, dark	1	1.6	55	2
rye, light, hard	1	1.0	79	2
sandwich	1	3.1	162	1
sesame seed	1	2.1	59	1
sourdough	1	1.0	100	1

Item	Serving	Total Fat (g)	Calories	Fiber (g)
submarine	1 medium	3.0	290	2
wheat	1	1.7	72	1
white, commercial	1	2.0	80	0
white, hmde	1	3.1	119	1
whole wheat	1	1.1	85	3
yeast, sweet	1	7.9	198	1
scone	1	5.5	120	1
soft pretzel	1 medium	1.7	190	1
stuffing				
bread, from mix	½ cup	12.2	198	0
cornbread, from mix	½ cup	4.8	175	0
Stove Top	½ cup	9.0	176	0
sweet roll, iced	1 medium	7.9	198	1
toaster pastry, any flavor	1	5.0	200	0
tortilla				
corn (unfried)	1 medium	1.1	67	1
flour	1 medium	2.5	85	1
turnover, fruit filled	1	15.0	280	1
waffle				
frozen	1 medium	3.2	95	1
hmde	1 large	12.6	245	1

Candy

butterscotch				
candy	6 pieces	1.3	140	0
chips	1 oz.	8.3	150	0
candied fruit				
apricot	1 oz.	0.1	94	1
cherry	1 oz.	0.1	96	1
citrus peel	1 oz.	0.1	90	1
figs	1 oz.	0.1	84	2
candy bar				
Almond Joy	1 oz.	7.8	136	2
Baby Ruth	1 oz.	6.6	141	1
Bit-O-Honey	1 oz.	2.2	121	0
Butterfinger	1 oz.	5.5	131	1
Chunky	1 oz.	8.3	140	1
Heath	1 oz.	8.9	142	1
Kit Kat	1.13 oz.	9.2	162	0
Mars	1.7 oz.	11.0	240	1

Item	Serving	Total Fat (g)	Calories	Fiber (g)
milk chocolate	1 oz.	9.2	147	1
milk choc. w/ almonds	1 oz.	10.1	151	2
Milky Way	1 oz.	4.3	120	0
Mounds	1 oz.	6.1	125	2
Mr. Goodbar	1 oz.	9.1	145	2
Nestlé Crunch	1.06 oz.	8.0	160	1
Snickers	1 oz.	6.5	135	1
Three Musketeers	1 oz.	3.7	120	0
Twix, caramel	1 oz.	6.7	140	0
candy-coated almonds	1 oz.	5.3	130	1
caramels				
plain or choc. w/ nuts	1 oz.	4.6	120	0
plain or choc. w/o nuts	1 oz.	3.0	110	0
carob-coated raisins	½ cup	13.5	387	5
choc. chips				
milk choc.	¼ cup	11.0	218	1
semi-sweet	¼ cup	12.2	220	1
choc.-covered cherries	1 oz.	4.9	123	1
choc.-covered cream center	1 oz.	4.9	123	1
choc.-covered mint patty	1 small	1.0	40	0
choc.-covered peanuts	1 oz.	11.7	159	2
choc.-covered raisins	1 oz.	4.9	120	1
choc. kisses	6 pieces	9.0	154	1
choc. stars	7 pieces	8.1	160	1
Cracker Jack	1 cup	3.3	170	2
English toffee	1 oz.	2.8	113	0
fondant	1 piece	0.2	116	0
fudge				
choc.	1 oz.	3.4	112	0
choc. w/ nuts	1 oz.	4.9	119	0
Good & Plenty	1 oz.	0.1	106	0
gumdrops	28 pieces	0.2	97	0
Gummy Bears	1 oz.	0.1	110	0
hard candy	6 pieces	0.3	108	0
jelly beans	1 oz.	0	104	0
licorice	1 oz.	0.1	35	0

Item	Serving	Total Fat (g)	Calories	Fiber (g)
M&Ms				
choc. only	1 oz.	5.6	132	1
peanut	1 oz.	7.8	145	1
malted-milk balls	1 oz.	7.1	137	1
marshmallow	1 large	0	25	0
marshmallow creme	1 oz.	0.1	88	0
mints	14 pieces	0.6	104	0
peanut brittle	1 oz.	7.7	149	1
Peanut Butter Cups, Reese's	1 oz.	9.2	156	1
Peppermint Pattie	1 oz.	4.8	124	1
praline	1 oz.	6.9	130	0
sour balls	1 oz.	0	110	0
taffy	1 oz.	1.5	99	0
Tootsie Roll pop	1 oz.	0.6	110	0
Tootsie Roll	1 oz.	2.3	112	1
yogurt-covered peanuts	½ cup	26.0	387	4
yogurt-covered raisins	½ cup	14.0	313	2

Cereals

Item	Serving	Total Fat (g)	Calories	Fiber (g)
All-Bran Bran Buds	⅓ cup	0.7	72	13
All-Bran Original	⅓ cup	0.5	70	10
Alpha-Bits	1 cup	0.6	111	1
Apple Jacks	1 cup	0.1	110	1
Bran, 100%	½ cup	1.9	84	9
bran, unprocessed, dry	¼ cup	0.6	29	6
Cap'n Crunch	¾ cup	1.5	110	1
Cheerios	1 cup	1.6	100	3
Cocoa Krispies	¾ cup	1.0	120	0
Corn Chex	1 cup	0.1	120	2
cornflakes	1 cup	0.1	108	1
corn grits w/o added fat	½ cup	0.5	71	1
Cream of Wheat w/o added fat	½ cup	0.3	67	1

Item	Serving	Total Fat (g)	Calories	Fiber (g)
Crispix	1 cup	0	110	1
Fiber One	1 cup	2.2	128	21
Frosted Flakes	1 cup	0.5	147	1
Frosted Mini-Wheats	4 biscuits	0.3	100	1
Golden Grahams	¾ cup	1.1	109	1
granola				
commercial brands	⅓ cup	4.9	126	3
hmde	⅓ cup	10.0	184	2
low-fat, Kellogg's	⅓ cup	2.0	120	2
Grape-Nuts	¼ cup	0.1	105	2
Grape-Nuts Flakes	1 cup	0.4	116	2
Honey Smacks	1 cup	0.7	140	1
Kix	1½ cup	0.7	110	0
Life, plain or cinn.	1 cup	2.5	152	4
Multi-Bran Chex	1 cup	1.2	136	9
Natural Bran Flakes	1 cup	0.7	127	9
oat bran, cooked cereal				
w/o added fat	½ cup	0.5	50	2
oat bran, dry	¼ cup	1.6	82	3
oats				
instant	1 packet	1.7	108	1
w/o added fat	½ cup	1.2	72	1
Product 19	1 cup	0.2	108	1
puffed rice	1 cup	0	56	0
puffed wheat	1 cup	0.1	44	1
Raisin Bran	1 cup	0.8	156	5
Rice Chex	1 cup	0.1	110	1
Rice Krispies	1 cup	0.2	110	0
shredded wheat	1 cup	1.0	170	6
Special K	1 cup	0.1	111	0
Total	1 cup	0.7	100	2
Total Raisin Bran	1 cup	1.0	140	5
Wheat Chex	1 cup	1.2	169	6

Item	Serving	Total Fat (g)	Calories	Fiber (g)
wheat germ, toasted	¼ cup	3.0	108	4
Wheaties	1 cup	0.5	99	2
whole-wheat, natural, w/o added fat	½ cup	0.5	75	2

Cheeses

Item	Serving	Total Fat (g)	Calories	Fiber (g)
American				
processed	1 oz.	8.9	106	0
reduced calorie	1 oz.	2.0	50	0
blue	1 oz.	8.2	100	0
brick	1 oz.	8.4	105	0
Brie	1 oz.	7.9	95	0
caraway	1 oz.	8.3	107	0
cheddar				
grated	¼ cup	9.4	114	0
sliced	1 oz.	9.4	114	0
cheese fondue	¼ cup	11.7	170	0
cheese food, cold pack	2 T	7.8	94	0
cheese sauce	¼ cup	9.8	132	0
cheese spread (Kraft)	1 oz.	6.0	82	0
Cheez Whiz	1 oz.	6.0	80	0
Colby	1 oz.	9.1	112	0
cottage cheese				
1% fat	½ cup	1.2	82	0
2% fat	½ cup	2.2	101	0
creamed	½ cup	5.1	117	0
cream cheese				
Kraft Free	1 oz. (2T)	0	25	0
"lite" (Neufchâtel)	1 oz. (2T)	6.6	74	0
regular	1 oz. (2T)	9.9	99	0
Edam	1 oz.	7.9	101	0
feta	1 oz.	6.0	75	0
Gouda	1 oz.	7.8	101	0
hot pepper cheese	1 oz.	6.9	92	0
Jarlsberg	1 oz.	6.9	100	0

Item	Serving	Total Fat (g)	Calories	Fiber (g)
Kraft American Singles	1 oz.	7.5	90	0
Limburger	1 oz.	7.7	93	0
Monterey Jack	1 oz.	8.6	106	0
mozzarella				
part skim	1 oz.	4.5	72	0
part skim, low moisture	1 oz.	4.9	79	0
whole milk	1 oz.	6.1	80	0
whole milk, low moisture	1 oz.	7.0	90	0
Muenster	1 oz.	8.5	104	0
Parmesan				
grated	1 T	1.5	23	0
hard	1 oz.	7.3	111	0
pimento cheese spread	1 oz.	8.9	106	0
port wine, cold pack	1 oz.	8.0	100	0
provolone	1 oz.	7.6	100	0
ricotta				
"lite" reduced fat	½ cup	4.0	109	0
part skim	½ cup	9.8	171	0
whole milk	½ cup	16.1	216	0
Romano	1 oz.	7.6	110	0
Roquefort	1 oz.	8.7	105	0
Sargento Reduced Fat				
mozzarella	1 oz.	4.5	80	0
Swiss	1 oz.	5.5	90	0
smoked cheese product	1 oz.	7.0	100	0
Swiss				
processed	1 oz.	7.1	95	0
sliced	1 oz.	7.8	107	0
Velveeta	1 oz.	7.0	100	0
Velveeta 2% milk	1 oz.	3.0	60	0
Weight Watchers, slices	1 oz.	2.0	50	0

Combination Foods

Item	Serving	Total Fat (g)	Calories	Fiber (g)
baked beans w/ pork	½ cup	1.8	134	4
beans				
refried, canned	½ cup	1.4	135	7

Item	Serving	Total Fat (g)	Calories	Fiber (g)
refried w/ fat	½ cup	13.2	271	7
refried w/ sausage, canned	½ cup	13.0	194	8
beans & franks, canned	1 cup	16.0	366	7
beef & vegetable stew	1 cup	10.5	218	2
beef goulash w/ noodles	1 cup	13.9	335	2
beef noodle casserole	1 cup	19.2	329	2
beef pot pie, frzn	8 oz.	23.0	430	2
beef stew, canned	1 cup	8.0	184	2
beef vegetable stew, hmde	1 cup	10.5	220	2
burrito				
bean w/ cheese	1 large	11.0	330	4
bean w/o cheese	1 large	6.8	225	4
beef	1 large	19.0	413	2
cabbage roll w/ beef & rice	1 medium	6.0	168	2
cannelloni, meat & cheese	1 piece	29.7	420	1
casserole, meat, veg., rice, sauce	1 cup	12.2	276	3
cheese soufflé	1 cup	14.1	195	0
chicken à la king, hmde	1 cup	34.3	468	1
chicken & dumplings	1 cup	10.5	298	1
chicken & rice casserole	1 cup	18.0	365	1
chicken & veg. stir-fry	1 cup	6.9	142	3
chicken divan, frzn	8½ oz.	22.2	353	1
chicken fricassee, hmde	1 cup	18.1	318	1
chicken-fried steak	3½ oz.	23.4	355	0
chicken noodle casserole	1 cup	10.7	269	2
chicken parmigiana, hmde	7 oz.	17.0	346	2
chicken pot pie, frzn	8 oz.	23.0	430	1
chicken salad, regular	½ cup	21.2	271	0
chicken tetrazzini	1 cup	19.6	348	1
chicken w/ cashews, Chinese	1 cup	28.6	409	2
chili				
w/ beans	1 cup	14.8	302	6
w/o beans	1 cup	19.3	302	3

Item	Serving	Total Fat (g)	Calories	Fiber (g)
chitterlings, cooked	3½ oz.	29.4	303	0
chop suey w/o rice or noodles				
beef	1 cup	15.8	275	2
fish or poultry	1 cup	8.2	195	2
chow mein				
beef, canned	1 cup	2.3	72	2
chicken, canned	1 cup	2.3	68	2
chicken, hmde	1 cup	8.8	224	2
corned-beef hash	1 cup	24.4	374	2
crab cake	1 small	4.5	95	0
creamed chipped beef	1 cup	23.0	350	0
curry w/o meat	1 cup	6.6	138	2
deviled crab	½ cup	15.4	231	1
deviled egg	1 large	5.3	63	0
egg foo yung w/ sauce	1 piece	7.0	129	1
eggplant parmigiana, traditional	1 cup	24.0	356	3
egg roll, restaurant style	1 (3½ oz.)	10.5	153	1
egg salad	½ cup	17.4	212	0
enchilada				
bean, beef, & cheese	1 piece	14.1	243	3
beef, frzn	7½ oz.	16.0	250	2
cheese, frzn	8 oz.	26.3	444	3
chicken, frzn	7½ oz.	16.1	340	4
fajitas				
chicken	1	13.5	381	4
beef	1	18.2	302	3
falafel	1 small	5.0	74	1
fettuccine Alfredo	1 cup	29.7	462	3
fish and chips, frzn dinner	5.5 oz.	14.8	325	3
fish creole	1 cup	5.4	172	2
fritter, corn	1 medium	8.5	132	1
frzn dinner				
beef tips and noodles	11 oz.	5.1	370	4
chopped sirloin	11.5 oz.	30.1	560	5
fried chicken	11 oz.	29.6	590	6
meat loaf	11 oz.	23.1	530	4

Item	Serving	Total Fat (g)	Calories	Fiber (g)
Salisbury steak	11 oz.	27.4	500	4
turkey and dressing	11 oz.	22.6	510	3
green pepper stuffed w/ rice & beef	1 average	13.5	262	2
Hamburger Helper, all varieties (average)	1 cup	18.9	375	1
hamburger rice casserole	1 cup	21.0	376	3
ham salad w/ mayo	½ cup	20.2	277	0
ham spread, Spreadables	½ cup	12.0	180	0
lasagna				
cheese, frzn	10½ oz.	14.0	390	5
hmde w/ beef & cheese	1 piece	19.8	400	2
zucchini lasagna, lo-cal, frzn	11 oz.	8.6	301	5
lobster				
Cantonese	1 cup	19.6	334	0
Newburg	½ cup	24.8	305	0
salad	½ cup	7.0	119	0
lo mein, Chinese	1 cup	7.2	185	1
macaroni & cheese				
from package	1 cup	17.3	386	0
frzn	6 oz.	12.0	260	0
manicotti, cheese & tomato	1 piece	11.8	238	2
meatball (reg. ground beef)	1 medium	5.1	72	0
meat loaf, w/ reg. ground beef	3½ oz.	20.4	332	0
moo goo gai pan	1 cup	17.2	304	1
moussaka	1 cup	8.9	210	3
onion rings	10 average	17.0	234	1
oysters Rockefeller, traditional	6–8 oysters	14.0	230	1
pepper steak	1 cup	11.0	330	1
pizza				
cheese	1 slice	10.1	270	1
combination w/ meat	1 slice	17.5	272	1
deep dish, cheese	1 slice	13.5	426	4
pepperoni, frzn	¼ pizza	18.0	364	2
pork, sweet & sour, w/ rice	1 cup	7.5	270	1

Item	Serving	Total Fat (g)	Calories	Fiber (g)
quiche				
Lorraine (bacon)	⅛ pie	43.5	540	1
plain or vegetable	1 slice	17.6	312	1
ratatouille	½ cup	3.0	60	2
ravioli, canned	1 cup	7.3	240	3
ravioli w/ meat & tomato sauce	1 piece	3.0	49	0
Salisbury steak w/ gravy	8 oz.	27.3	364	1
salmon patty, traditional	3½ oz.	12.4	239	1
sandwiches (on white bread unless otherwise noted)				
BBQ beef on bun	1	16.8	392	5
BBQ pork on bun	1	12.2	359	5
BLT w/ mayo	1	15.6	282	2
bologna & cheese	1	22.5	363	2
chicken w/ mayo & lettuce	1	14.4	303	2
club w/ mayo	1	20.8	590	3
corned beef on rye	1	10.8	296	2
egg salad	1	12.5	279	2
french dip, au jus	1	12.2	360	2
grilled cheese	1	24.0	426	2
ham, cheese & mayo	1	16.0	350	2
ham salad	1	16.9	321	2
peanut butter & jelly	1	15.1	374	3
Reuben	1	33.3	531	6
roast beef & mayo	1	22.6	328	2
sloppy joe on bun	1	16.8	392	5
sub w/ salami & cheese	1	41.3	766	3
tuna salad	1	17.5	362	2
turkey & mayo	1	18.4	402	2
turkey breast & mustard	1	5.2	285	2
turkey ham on rye	1	10.5	239	3
shepherd's pie	1 cup	24.0	407	3
shrimp creole w/o rice	1 cup	6.1	146	2
shrimp salad	½ cup	9.5	136	1
spaghetti				
w/ meat sauce	1 cup	16.7	317	2
w/ red clam sauce	1 cup	7.3	250	2
w/ tomato sauce	1 cup	1.5	179	2
w/ white clam sauce	1 cup	19.5	416	1

Item	Serving	Total Fat (g)	Calories	Fiber (g)
spanakopita	1 piece	24.1	259	2
spinach soufflé	1 cup	14.8	212	2
stroganoff				
beef w/ noodles	1 cup	19.6	390	2
beef w/o noodles	1 cup	26.8	460	1
sushi w/ fish & vegetables	5 oz.	1.0	210	1
taco, beef	1 medium	17.0	272	2
tamale w/ sauce	1 piece	6.0	114	1
tortellini, meat or cheese	1 cup	15.4	363	1
tostada w/ refried beans	1 medium	16.3	294	6
tuna noodle casserole	1 cup	13.3	315	2
tuna salad				
oil pack, w/ mayo	½ cup	16.3	226	0
water pack, w/ mayo	½ cup	10.5	170	0
veal parmigiana, hmde	1 cup	25.5	485	2
veal scallopini	1 cup	20.4	429	2
Welsh rarebit	1 cup	31.6	415	0
wonton w/ pork, fried	1 piece	4.3	82	0
Yorkshire pudding	1 piece	2.4	56	0

Desserts and Toppings

Item	Serving	Total Fat (g)	Calories	Fiber (g)
apple betty, fruit crisps	½ cup	13.3	347	3
baklava	1 piece	29.2	426	2
brownie				
butterscotch	1	6.6	150	0
choc., "light," from mix	¹⁄₂₄ pkg.	2.0	100	0
choc., plain	1	1.5	64	0
choc., w/ frosting	1	9.0	210	1
choc., w/ nuts	1	7.3	170	1
cake				
angel food	¹⁄₁₂ cake	0.1	161	0
banana w/ frosting	¹⁄₁₂ cake	16.0	410	1
black forest	¹⁄₁₂ cake	14.3	279	1
butter w/ frosting	¹⁄₁₂ cake	13.0	380	1
carrot w/ frosting	¹⁄₁₂ cake	19.0	420	3
choc. w/ frosting	¹⁄₁₂ cake	17.0	388	2
coconut w/ frosting	¹⁄₁₂ cake	18.1	395	2

Item	Serving	Total Fat (g)	Calories	Fiber (g)
devil's food, "light," from mix	1/12 cake	3.5	190	0
German choc. w/ frosting	1/12 cake	18.5	407	2
gingerbread	2½" slice	2.9	267	0
lemon chiffon	1/12 cake	4.0	190	0
lemon w/ frosting	1/12 cake	16.0	410	1
pineapple upside-down	2½" slice	9.1	236	2
pound	1/12 cake	9.0	200	1
shortbread w/ fruit	1 piece	8.9	344	1
spice w/ frosting	1/12 cake	11.3	375	1
sponge	1 piece	3.1	190	0
white w/ frosting	1/12 cake	14.6	369	1
white, "light," from mix	1/12 cake	3.0	180	0
yellow, "light," from mix	1/12 cake	3.5	190	0
yellow w/ frosting	1/12 cake	16.4	391	1
cheesecake, traditional	1/8 pie	22.0	372	0
cobbler				
w/ biscuit topping	½ cup	6.0	209	3
w/ pie-crust topping	½ cup	9.3	236	3
cookie				
animal	15 cookies	4.7	152	0
anise-seed	1	4.0	63	0
anisette toast	1 slice	1.0	109	0
arrowroot	1	0.9	24	0
choc.	1	3.3	56	0
choc. chip, hmde	1	3.7	68	0
choc. chip, Pepperidge Farm	1	2.5	100	0
choc. sandwich (Oreo type)	1	2.1	49	0
fig bar	1	1.0	56	1
gingersnap	1	1.6	34	0
graham cracker, choc. covered	1	3.1	62	0
macaroon, coconut	1	3.4	60	0
molasses	1	3.0	80	0
oatmeal	1	3.2	80	0
oatmeal raisin	1	3.0	83	0
peanut butter	1	3.2	72	1
Rice Krispie bar	1	0.9	36	0
shortbread	1	2.3	42	0
sugar	1	3.4	89	0
sugar wafers	2 small	2.1	53	0
vanilla-creme sandwich	1	3.1	69	0
vanilla wafers	3	1.8	51	0
cream puff w/ custard	1	14.6	245	0

Item	Serving	Total Fat (g)	Calories	Fiber (g)
cupcake				
choc. w/ icing	1	5.5	159	1
yellow w/ icing	1	6.0	160	1
custard, baked	½ cup	6.9	148	0
date bar	1 bar	2.0	90	1
dumpling, fruit	1 piece	15.1	324	2
eclair				
w/ choc. icing & custard	1 small	15.4	316	0
w/ choc. icing & whipped				
cream	1 small	25.7	296	0
frosting/icing				
choc.	3 T	5.3	148	0
cream cheese	3 T	6.8	170	0
"light" varieties, ready-to-				
spread	1⁄12 tub	2.0	130	0
ready-to-spread	1⁄12 tub	6.9	169	0
seven-minute	3 T	0	135	0
vanilla or lemon	3 T	4.0	140	0
fruitcake	1 piece	6.2	154	1
fruit ice, Italian	½ cup	0	123	0
Fudgsicle	1 bar	0.4	196	1
gelatin				
low-cal.	½ cup	0	8	0
regular, sweetened	½ cup	0	70	0
granola bar	1 bar	6.8	141	1
Hostess				
brownie	1	12.0	350	1
cupcake	1	5.0	170	1
cupcake lights	1	1.5	120	0
Ding Dong	1	9.0	160	0
fruit snack pie	1	14.4	266	2
Ho Ho	1	6.0	120	1
honey bun	1	23.0	410	2
Snoball	1	4.0	150	1
Twinkie	1	4.0	140	0
Twinkie lights	1	1.5	120	0
ice cream				
choc. (10% fat)	½ cup	7.3	145	1
choc. (16% fat)	½ cup	17.0	270	0
dietetic, sugar free	½ cup	3.5	90	0

Item	Serving	Total Fat (g)	Calories	Fiber (g)
strawberry (10% fat)	½ cup	6.0	128	0
vanilla (10% fat)	½ cup	7.2	134	0
vanilla (16% fat)	½ cup	11.9	175	0
ice cream bar				
choc. coated	1 bar	11.5	198	0
toffee krunch	1 bar	10.2	149	1
ice cream cake roll	1 slice	6.9	159	0
ice cream cone (cone only)	1 medium	0.3	45	0
ice cream drumstick	1	10.0	188	1
ice cream sandwich	1	8.3	204	0
ice milk				
choc.	½ cup	2.0	100	0
soft serve, all flavors	½ cup	2.3	112	0
strawberry	½ cup	2.5	100	0
vanilla	½ cup	2.8	92	0
ladyfinger	1	2.0	60	0
lemon bars	1 bar	3.2	70	0
mousse, choc.	½ cup	15.5	189	1
napoleon	1 piece	5.3	85	0
pie				
apple	⅛ pie	16.9	347	3
banana cream or custard	⅛ pie	14.0	353	1
blueberry	⅛ pie	17.3	387	3
Boston cream	⅛ pie	10.0	302	1
cherry	⅛ pie	18.1	418	2
choc. cream	⅛ pie	13.0	311	3
choc. meringue, traditional	⅛ pie	18.0	378	1
coconut cream or custard	⅛ pie	19.0	365	1
key lime	⅛ pie	19.0	388	1
lemon chiffon	⅛ pie	13.5	335	1
lemon meringue, traditional	⅛ pie	13.1	350	1
mincemeat	⅛ pie	18.4	434	3
peach	⅛ pie	17.7	421	3
pecan	⅛ pie	23.0	510	2
pumpkin	⅛ pie	16.8	367	5
raisin	⅛ pie	12.9	325	1
rhubarb	⅛ pie	17.1	405	3
strawberry	⅛ pie	9.1	228	1
sweet potato	⅛ pie	18.2	342	2

Item	Serving	Total Fat (g)	Calories	Fiber (g)
pie tart, fruit filled	1	18.7	362	2
Popsicle	1 bar	0	96	0
pudding				
any flavor except choc.	½ cup	4.3	165	0
bread w/ raisins	½ cup	7.4	212	1
choc. w/ whole milk	½ cup	5.7	220	1
from mix w/ skim milk	½ cup	0	124	0
noodle	½ cup	5.3	141	0
rice, w/ whole milk	½ cup	4.4	170	1
sugar-free varieties	½ cup	2.2	90	0
tapioca, w/ 2% milk	½ cup	2.4	150	0
pudding pop, frzn	1 bar	2.0	80	0
sherbet	½ cup	1.0	130	0
sopaipilla	1 piece	6.0	88	0
soufflé, choc	½ cup	3.9	63	0
strudel, fruit	½ cup	1.2	47	1
toppings				
butterscotch/caramel	3 T	0.1	156	0
cherry	3 T	0.1	147	0
choc. fudge	2 T	4.0	110	1
choc. syrup, Hershey	2 T	0.4	73	1
custard sauce, hmde	3 T	2.9	64	0
lemon sauce, hmde	3 T	2.1	100	0
marshmallow creme	3 T	0	158	0
pecans in syrup	3 T	2.8	168	0
pineapple	3 T	0.2	146	0
raisin sauce, hmde	3 T	3.0	126	0
strawberry	3 T	0.1	139	0
whipped topping				
aerosol	¼ cup	3.6	45	0
from mix	¼ cup	2.0	32	0
frzn, tub	¼ cup	4.8	59	0
"lite"	1 T	0.3	5	0
whipping cream				
heavy, fluid	1 T	5.6	52	0
light, fluid	1 T	4.6	44	0
turnover, fruit filled	1	19.3	226	1
yogurt, frozen				
low fat	½ cup	1.9	120	0
nonfat	½ cup	0.2	100	0

Item	Serving	Total Fat (g)	Calories	Fiber (g)
Eggs				
boiled-poached	1	5.6	79	0
fried w/ ½ t fat	1 large	7.8	104	0
omelet				
2 oz. cheese, 3 egg	1	37.0	510	0
plain, 3 egg	1	21.3	271	0
scrambled w/ milk	1 large	8.0	101	0
substitute	¼ cup	0	30	0
white	1 large	0	17	0
yolk	1 large	5.6	63	0
Fast Food				
Arby's				
Arby's Melt	1	16.0	390	2
Ham & Swiss Melt	1	8.0	300	2
potato cakes	2 pieces	15.0	260	2
Roast Beef Classic	1	14.0	360	2
Roast Chicken Club	1	18.0	460	2
Burger King				
cheeseburger	1	19.0	380	1
french fries, medium	1 order	17.0	370	4
hamburger	1	16.0	340	1
Whopper	1	39.0	680	3
Whopper w/ cheese	1	47.0	780	3
Domino's Pizza				
Deep Dish, cheese only				
14" pizza	1 slice	16.0	350	4
Hand Tossed, cheese only				
14" pizza	1 slice	11.0	290	2
Thin Crust, cheese only				
14" pizza	1 slice	11.5	290	2
KFC				
Crispy Strips	3 pieces	21.0	390	0
grilled chicken breast	1	7.0	220	0
grilled chicken thigh	1	10.0	170	0
Hot Wings	1	4.0	70	0
Original Recipe chicken breast	1	21.0	360	0
Original Recipe chicken thigh	1	17.0	250	0

Item	Serving	Total Fat (g)	Calories	Fiber (g)
McDonald's				
baked apple pie	1	13.0	250	4
bacon, egg, & cheese biscuit	1	23.0	420	2
Big Mac	1	29.0	540	3
cheeseburger	1	12.0	300	2
Chicken McNuggets	4 pieces	12.0	190	1
Chipotle BBQ Snack Wrap (grilled)	1	9.0	260	1
Egg McMuffin	1	12.0	300	2
french fries, medium	1 order	19.0	380	5
Fruit & Maple Oatmeal	1	4.5	290	5
hamburger	1	9.0	250	2
Premium Caesar salad	1	4.0	90	3
Quarter Pounder	1	19.0	410	3
Quarter Pounder w/ cheese	1	26.0	510	3
Pizza Hut				
cheese pizza, 14"				
classic	1 slice	10.0	260	1
pan	1 slice	12.0	270	1
stuffed crust	1 slice	22.0	490	2
Thin 'N Crispy	1 slice	9.0	230	1
Subway				
6-inch sub sandwiches on 9-grain wheat bread				
Fresh Fit Choices				
Black Forest Ham	1	4.5	290	5
Oven Roasted Chicken	1	5.0	320	5
Roast Beef	1	5.0	320	5
Subway Club	1	4.5	310	5
Turkey Breast	1	3.5	280	5
Turkey Melt	1	7.0	320	5
Veggie Delite	1	2.5	230	5
Hot and Fresh Toasted				
Big Philly Cheesesteak	1	18.0	520	6
Chicken & Bacon Ranch	1	28.0	570	5
Meatball Marinara	1	23.0	570	9
Spicy Italian	1	28.0	520	5
Subway Melt	1	11.0	370	5
Taco Bell				
burritos				
bean	1	10.0	370	10
Burrito Supremo, beef	1	15.0	420	9
Burrito Supremo, chicken	1	12.0	400	12
grilled chicken	1	18.0	430	3

Item	Serving	Total Fat (g)	Calories	Fiber (g)
specialties				
MexiMelt	1	14.0	270	4
Enchirito, beef	1	17.0	460	8
Express Taco Salad w/ chips	1	28.0	580	9
Tostada	1	10.0	250	9
Mexican Pizza	1	30.0	540	8
tacos				
crunchy taco	1	10.0	170	3
Fresco Chicken soft taco	1	3.5	150	2
Grilled Steak soft taco	1	14.0	250	2
soft taco, beef	1	9.0	210	3
Wendy's				
chili, small	1	6.0	210	6
Crispy Chicken sandwich	1	16.0	350	2
french fries, medium	1 order	21.0	420	6
Grilled Chicken Go Wrap	1	10.0	260	1
hamburger, single, ¼ pound	1	28.0	550	2
Junior cheeseburger	1	11.0	270	1
Junior hamburger	1	8.0	230	1
Original chocolate frosty, medium	1	9.0	340	0
Fats				
bacon fat	1 T	14.0	126	0
beef, separable fat	1 oz.	23.3	216	0
butter				
solid	1 t	3.8	34	0
whipped	1 t	2.6	23	0
cream				
light	1 T	2.9	29	0
medium (25% fat)	1 T	3.8	37	0
whipping, light	1 T	4.6	44	0
cream substitute				
liquid/frzn	½ fl. oz.	1.5	20	0
powdered	1 T	0.7	11	0
half & half	1 T	1.7	20	0
margarine				
liquid or soft tub	1 t	3.8	34	0
reduced calorie, tub	1 t	2.0	18	0
solid (corn), stick	1 t	3.8	34	0

Item	Serving	Total Fat (g)	Calories	Fiber (g)
mayonnaise				
fat free	1 T	0	11	0
reduced calorie	1 T	5.0	50	0
regular (soybean)	1 T	11.0	100	0
no-stick spray				
(Pam, etc.)	2-sec spray	0.9	8	0
oil				
canola	1 T	13.6	120	0
corn	1 T	13.6	120	0
olive	1 T	13.5	119	0
safflower	1 T	13.6	120	0
soybean	1 T	13.6	120	0
pork				
backfat, raw	1 oz.	25.4	192	0
separable fat, cooked	1 oz.	23.4	216	0
pork fat (lard)	1 T	12.8	116	0
salt pork, raw	1 oz.	23.8	219	0
sandwich spread (Miracle Whip type)	1 T	4.9	57	0
shortening, vegetable	1 T	12.8	113	0
sour cream				
cultured	1 T	3.0	31	0
fat free	1 T	0	9	0
half & half, cultured	1 T	1.8	20	0
imitation	1 T	2.8	30	0
"lite"	1 T	1.8	20	0
Fish (all baked/broiled w/o added fat unless otherwise noted)				
abalone, canned	3½ oz.	5.6	80	0
anchovy, canned in oil	3 fillets	1.2	25	0
anchovy paste	1 t	0.8	14	0
bass				
freshwater	3½ oz.	4.7	145	0
saltwater, black	3½ oz.	1.2	93	0
saltwater, striped	3½ oz.	2.5	105	0
bluefish	3½ oz.	5.4	157	0

Item	Serving	Total Fat (g)	Calories	Fiber (g)
buffalo fish	3½ oz.	4.2	150	0
butterfish				
gulf	3½ oz.	2.9	95	0
northern	3½ oz.	10.2	184	0
carp	3½ oz.	6.1	138	0
catfish	3½ oz.	3.1	103	0
catfish, breaded & fried	3½ oz.	13.2	226	NA
caviar, sturgeon, granular	1 round t	1.5	26	0
clams				
canned, solids & liquid	½ cup	0.7	85	0
canned, solids only	3 oz.	1.6	118	0
meat only	5 large	1.0	80	0
cod				
canned	3½ oz.	0.8	104	0
cooked	3½ oz.	0.8	104	0
dried, salted	3½ oz.	2.3	287	0
crab				
canned	½ cup	0.9	67	0
deviled	3½ oz.	10.1	217	0
crab, Alaska king	3½ oz.	1.5	96	0
crab cake	3½ oz.	10.8	178	0
crappie, white	3½ oz.	0.8	79	0
crayfish, freshwater	3½ oz.	1.4	89	0
crooker				
Atlantic	3½ oz.	3.2	133	0
white	3½ oz.	0.8	84	0
cusk, steamed	3½ oz.	0.9	111	0
dolphinfish	3½ oz.	0.8	93	0
eel, American				
cooked	3½ oz.	18.3	260	0
smoked	3½ oz.	23.6	281	0
eulachon (smelt)	3½ oz.	6.2	118	0
fillets, frzn				
batter dipped	2 pieces	20.0	340	1
breaded	2 pieces	18.0	290	1
fish cakes, frzn, fried	3½ oz.	14.0	242	2
flatfish	3½ oz.	0.8	79	0

Item	Serving	Total Fat (g)	Calories	Fiber (g)
flounder/sole	3½ oz.	0.5	68	0
gefilte fish	3½ oz.	2.2	82	1
grouper	3½ oz.	1.3	87	0
haddock				
cooked	3½ oz.	0.6	79	0
fried	3½ oz.	14.2	284	0
smoked/canned	3½ oz.	0.4	103	0
halibut	3½ oz.	1.2	100	0
herring				
canned or smoked	3½ oz.	13.6	208	0
cooked	3½ oz.	11.3	176	0
pickled	3½ oz.	15.1	223	0
Jack mackerel	3½ oz.	5.6	143	0
kingfish	3½ oz.	3.0	105	0
lobster, northern				
broiled w/ fat	12 oz.	15.1	445	0
cooked	3½ oz.	0.6	97	0
mackerel				
Atlantic	3½ oz.	13.7	204	0
Pacific	3½ oz.	7.3	159	0
muskellunge				
("muskie," "skie")	3½ oz.	2.5	109	0
mussels, meat only	3½ oz.	2.2	95	0
ocean perch				
cooked	3½ oz.	1.6	95	0
fried	3½ oz.	11.6	228	0
octopus	3½ oz.	2.1	163	0
oysters				
canned	3½ oz.	2.2	76	0
fried	3½ oz.	13.9	239	0
raw	5–8 medium	1.8	66	0
perch, freshwater, yellow	3½ oz.	0.9	91	0
pickerel	3½ oz.	0.5	84	0
pike				
blue	3½ oz.	0.9	90	0
northern	3½ oz.	1.1	88	0
walleye	3½ oz.	1.2	93	0

Item	Serving	Total Fat (g)	Calories	Fiber (g)
pollock, Atlantic	3½ oz.	1.0	91	0
pompano	3½ oz.	9.5	166	0
rainbow trout				
baked, broiled	3½ oz.	5.8	150	0
breaded, fried	3½ oz.	14.6	265	1
red snapper	3½ oz.	1.9	93	0
rockfish, oven steamed	3½ oz.	2.5	107	0
roughy, orange	3½ oz.	7.0	124	0
salmon				
Atlantic	3½ oz.	6.3	141	0
broiled/baked	3½ oz.	7.4	182	0
chinook, canned	3½ oz.	14.0	210	0
pink, canned	3½ oz.	5.1	118	0
smoked	3½ oz.	9.3	176	0
sardines				
Atlantic, in soy oil	2 sardines	2.8	50	0
Pacific	3½ oz.	8.6	160	0
scallops				
cooked	3½ oz.	1.2	81	0
frzn, fried	3½ oz.	10.5	194	0
steamed	3½ oz.	1.4	112	0
sea bass, white	3½ oz.	1.5	96	0
shrimp				
canned, dry pack	3½ oz.	1.6	116	0
canned, wet pack	½ cup	0.8	87	0
fried	3½ oz.	10.8	225	0
raw or broiled	3½ oz.	1.8	105	0
smelt	3½ oz.	2.4	100	0
sole, fillet	3½ oz.	0.5	68	0
squid				
fried	3 oz.	6.4	149	0
raw	3 oz.	1.2	78	0
surimi	3½ oz.	0.9	98	0
sushi or sashimi	3½ oz.	4.9	144	0
swordfish	3½ oz.	4.0	118	0
trout				
brook	3½ oz.	2.1	101	0
rainbow	3½ oz.	11.4	195	0

Item	Serving	Total Fat (g)	Calories	Fiber (g)
tuna				
albacore, raw	3½ oz.	7.5	177	0
bluefin, raw	3½ oz.	4.1	145	0
canned, light in oil	3½ oz.	8.1	197	0
canned, light in water	3½ oz.	0.8	115	0
canned, white in oil	3½ oz.	8.0	185	0
canned, white in water	3½ oz.	2.4	135	0
yellowfin, raw	3½ oz.	3.0	133	0
white perch	3½ oz.	3.9	114	0
whiting	3½ oz.	1.7	114	0
yellowtail	3½ oz.	5.4	138	0

Fruit

Item	Serving	Total Fat (g)	Calories	Fiber (g)
apple				
dried	½ cup	0.1	155	5
whole w/ peel	1 medium	0.4	81	4
applesauce, unsweetened	½ cup	0.1	53	2
apricots				
dried	5 halves	0.2	83	6
fresh	3 medium	0.4	51	2
avocado				
California	1 (6 oz.)	30.0	306	4
Florida	1 (11 oz.)	27.0	339	4
banana	1 medium	0.6	105	2
banana chips	½ cup	15.5	240	4
blackberries				
fresh	1 cup	0.6	74	7
frzn, unsweetened	1 cup	0.7	97	7
blueberries				
fresh	1 cup	0.6	82	5
frzn, unsweetened	1 cup	0.7	80	4
boysenberries, frzn unsweetened	1 cup	0.4	66	6
breadfruit, fresh	¼ small	0.2	99	3
cantaloupe	1 cup	0.4	57	3
cherries				
maraschino	¼ cup	0.2	66	1

Item	Serving	Total Fat (g)	Calories	Fiber (g)
sour, canned in heavy syrup	½ cup	0.1	116	1
sweet	½ cup	0.7	49	2
cranberries, fresh	1 cup	0.2	46	4
cranberry-orange relish	½ cup	0.9	246	3
cranberry sauce	½ cup	0.2	209	1
dates, whole, dried	½ cup	0.4	228	8
figs				
canned	3 figs	0.1	75	9
dried, uncooked	10 figs	1.1	254	10
fresh	1 medium	0.2	37	2
fruit cocktail, canned w/ juice	1 cup	0.3	112	5
grapefruit	½ medium	0.1	39	1
grapes, Thompson seedless	½ cup	0.1	94	1
guava, fresh	1 medium	0.5	45	7
honeydew melon, fresh	¼ small	0.1	46	1
kiwi, fresh	1 medium	0.3	46	2
kumquat, fresh	1 medium	0	12	1
lemon, fresh	1 medium	0.2	17	1
lime, fresh	1 medium	0.1	20	1
mandarin oranges, canned w/ juice	½ cup	0	46	4
mango, fresh	1 medium	0.6	135	4
melon balls, frzn	1 cup	0.4	55	2
mixed fruit				
dried	½ cup	0.5	243	6
frzn, sweetened	1 cup	0.5	245	2
mulberries, fresh	1 cup	0.6	61	3
nectarine, fresh	1 medium	0.6	67	2
orange	1 medium	0.1	65	4
papaya, fresh	1 medium	0.4	117	3
passionfruit, purple, fresh	1 medium	0.1	18	3
peach				
canned in heavy syrup	1 cup	0.3	190	4
canned in light syrup	1 cup	0.1	136	4

Item	Serving	Total Fat (g)	Calories	Fiber (g)
fresh	1 medium	0.1	37	1
frzn, sweetened	1 cup	0.3	235	4
pear				
canned in heavy syrup	1 cup	0.3	188	6
canned in light syrup	1 cup	0.1	144	6
fresh	1 medium	0.7	98	5
persimmon, fresh	1 medium	0.1	32	3
pineapple pieces				
canned, unsweetened	1 cup	0.2	150	2
fresh	1 cup	0.7	77	3
plantain, cooked, sliced	1 cup	0.3	179	1
plum				
canned in heavy syrup	½ cup	0.1	119	4
fresh	1 medium	0.4	36	3
pomegranate, fresh	1 medium	0.5	104	2
prickly pear, fresh	1 medium	0.5	42	3
prunes, dried, cooked	½ cup	0.2	113	10
raisins				
dark seedless	¼ cup	0.2	112	3
golden seedless	¼ cup	0.2	113	3
raspberries				
fresh	1 cup	0.7	61	6
frzn, sweetened	1 cup	0.4	256	12
rhubarb, stewed, unsweetened	1 cup	0.2	26	6
star fruit/carambola	1 medium	0.4	42	2
strawberries				
fresh	1 cup	0.6	45	3
frzn, sweetened	1 cup	0.3	245	3
frzn, unsweetened	1 cup	0.2	52	3
sugar apples, fresh	1 medium	0.5	146	4
tangelo, fresh	1 medium	0.1	39	3
tangerine, fresh	1 medium	0.2	37	3
watermelon, fresh	1 cup	0.5	50	1

Fruit Juices and Nectars

apple juice	1 cup	0.3	116	0

Item	Serving	Total Fat (g)	Calories	Fiber (g)
apricot nectar	1 cup	0.2	141	2
carrot juice	1 cup	0.4	97	2
cranberry juice cocktail				
low cal	1 cup	0	45	0
regular	1 cup	0.2	144	0
cranberry-apple juice	1 cup	0.2	170	0
grape juice	1 cup	0.2	128	1
grapefruit juice	1 cup	0.2	93	0
lemon juice	2 T	0	6	0
lime juice	2 T	0	6	0
orange juice	1 cup	0.4	105	1
orange-grapefruit juice	1 cup	0.2	107	1
peach juice or nectar	1 cup	0.1	134	1
pear juice or nectar	1 cup	0	149	1
pineapple juice	1 cup	0.2	139	1
pineapple-orange juice	1 cup	0.1	125	1
prune juice	1 cup	0.1	181	3
tomato juice	1 cup	0.2	43	2
V8 juice	1 cup	0.1	49	2
Gravies, Sauces, and Dips				
au jus, mix	½ cup	0.7	16	0
barbecue sauce	1 T	0.3	12	0
béarnaise sauce, mix	¼ pkg.	25.6	263	0
beef gravy, canned	½ cup	2.8	62	0
brown gravy				
from mix	½ cup	0.9	38	0
hmde	¼ cup	14.0	164	0
chicken gravy				
canned	½ cup	6.8	95	0
from mix	½ cup	0.9	42	0
giblet, hmde	¼ cup	2.6	49	0
chili sauce	1 T	0	18	0
dip made with sour cream	2 T	6.0	67	0

Item	Serving	Total Fat (g)	Calories	Fiber (g)
guacamole dip	1 oz.	4.0	50	0
hollandaise sauce	¼ cup	18.0	170	0
home-style gravy, from mix	¼ cup	0.5	25	0
jalapeño dip	1 oz.	1.1	33	0
ketchup, tomato	1 T	0.1	16	0
mushroom gravy				
canned	½ cup	3.2	60	1
from mix	½ cup	0.4	35	1
mushroom sauce, from mix	¼ pkg.	0.7	25	0
mustard				
brown	1 T	1.8	26	1
yellow	1 T	0.7	12	0
onion dip	2 T	6.0	67	0
onion gravy, from mix	½ cup	0.4	39	0
pesto sauce	½ cup	29.0	310	1
picante sauce	½ cup	0.8	53	2
pork gravy, from mix	½ cup	1.0	38	0
sour-cream sauce	¼ cup	7.6	128	0
soy sauce	1 T	0	10	0
soy sauce, reduced sodium	1 T	0	10	0
spaghetti sauce				
"healthy"/"lite" varieties	½ cup	1.0	60	3
hmde, w/ ground beef	½ cup	8.3	145	2
marinara	½ cup	4.7	95	3
meat flavor, jar	½ cup	6.0	100	2
meatless, jar	½ cup	2.0	70	2
mushroom, jar	½ cup	2.0	70	2
spinach dip (sour cream & mayo)	2 T	7.1	74	1
steak sauce				
A1	1 T	0	10	0
others	1 T	0	18	0
stroganoff sauce, mix	¼ pkg.	2.9	73	0
sweet & sour sauce	¼ cup	0.1	60	0
Tabasco sauce	1 t	0	1	0
taco sauce	1 T	0	5	0

Item	Serving	Total Fat (g)	Calories	Fiber (g)
tartar sauce	1 T	8.2	74	0
teriyaki sauce	1 T	0	15	0
turkey gravy				
canned	½ cup	2.4	58	0
from mix	½ cup	0.9	43	0
white sauce	¼ cup	6.8	90	0
Worcestershire sauce	1 T	0	10	0
Meats *(all cooked w/o added fat unless otherwise noted)*				
beef, extra lean, < 5% fat by weight (cooked)				
round, eye of, lean	3½ oz.	4.2	155	0
beef, lean, 5–10.4% fat by weight (cooked)				
arm/blade, lean pot roast	3½ oz.	9.4	207	0
flank steak, fat trimmed	3½ oz.	8.0	193	0
hindshank, lean	3½ oz.	9.4	207	0
porterhouse steak, lean	3½ oz.	10.4	225	0
rib steak, lean	3½ oz.	9.4	207	0
round				
bottom, lean	3½ oz.	9.4	207	0
roasted	3½ oz.	7.4	189	0
rump, lean, pot-roasted	3½ oz.	7.0	179	0
top, lean	3½ oz.	6.4	211	0
short plate, sep. lean only	3½ oz.	10.4	225	0
sirloin steak, lean	3½ oz.	8.9	201	0
sirloin tip, lean roasted	3½ oz.	9.4	207	0
tenderloin, lean, broiled	3½ oz.	11.1	219	0
top sirloin, lean, broiled	3½ oz.	7.9	201	0
beef, regular, 10.5–17.4% fat by weight (cooked)				
chuck, separable lean	3½ oz.	15.2	268	0
club steak, lean	3½ oz.	12.9	240	0
cubed steak	3½ oz.	15.4	264	0
hamburger				
extra lean	3 oz.	13.9	253	0
lean	3 oz.	15.7	268	0
rib roast, lean	3½ oz.	15.2	264	0
sirloin tips, roasted	3½ oz.	15.2	264	0
stew meat, round, raw	4 oz.	15.3	294	0

Item	Serving	Total Fat (g)	Calories	Fiber (g)
T-bone, lean only	3½ oz.	10.3	212	0
tenderloin, marbled	3½ oz.	15.2	264	0
beef, high fat,—17.5–27.4% fat by weight (cooked)				
arm/blade, pot-roasted	3½ oz.	26.5	354	0
chuck, ground	3½ oz.	23.9	327	0
hamburger, regular	3 oz.	19.6	286	0
meatballs	1 oz.	5.5	78	0
porterhouse steak, lean & marbled	3½ oz.	19.6	286	0
rib steak	3½ oz.	14.7	286	0
rump, pot-roasted	3½ oz.	19.6	286	0
short ribs, lean	3½ oz.	19.6	286	0
sirloin, broiled	3½ oz.	18.7	278	0
sirloin, ground	3½ oz.	26.5	354	0
T-bone, broiled	3½ oz.	26.5	354	0
beef, highest fat, ≥ 27.5% fat by weight (cooked)				
brisket, lean & marbled	3½ oz.	30.0	367	0
chuck, stew meat	3½ oz.	30.0	367	0
corned, medium fat	3½ oz.	30.2	372	0
ribeye steak, marbled	3½ oz.	38.8	440	0
rib roast	3½ oz.	30.0	367	0
short ribs	3½ oz.	31.7	382	0
steak, chicken fried	3½ oz.	30.0	389	0
lamb				
blade chop				
lean	1 chop	6.4	128	0
lean & marbled	3½ oz.	26.1	380	0
leg				
lean	3½ oz.	8.1	180	0
lean & marbled	3½ oz.	14.5	242	0
loin chop				
lean	3½ oz.	8.1	180	0
lean & marbled	3½ oz.	22.5	302	0
rib chop				
lean	3½ oz.	8.1	180	0
lean & marbled	3½ oz.	21.2	292	0
shoulder				
lean	3½ oz.	9.9	248	0
lean & marbled	3½ oz.	27.0	430	0
miscellaneous meats				
bacon substitute (breakfast strip)	2 strips	4.8	50	0

Item	Serving	Total Fat (g)	Calories	Fiber (g)
beefalo	3½ oz.	6.3	188	0
frog legs				
cooked	4 large	0.3	73	0
flour coated & fried	6 large	28.6	418	0
rabbit, stewed	3½ oz.	10.1	216	0
venison, roasted	3½ oz.	2.5	157	0
organ meats				
brains, all kinds, raw	3 oz.	7.4	106	0
heart				
beef, lean, braised	3½ oz.	5.6	175	0
kidney, beef, braised	3½ oz.	3.4	144	0
liver				
beef, braised	3½ oz.	4.9	161	0
beef, pan fried	3½ oz.	8.0	217	0
calf, braised	3½ oz.	6.9	165	0
calf, pan fried	3½ oz.	11.4	245	0
tongue				
beef, etc., pickled	1 oz.	5.8	76	0
beef, etc., potted	1 oz.	6.6	83	0
beef, med. fat, simmered	3 oz.	17.6	241	0
pork				
bacon				
cured, broiled	1 strip	3.1	35	0
cured, raw	1 oz.	16.3	158	0
blade				
lean	3½ oz.	9.6	219	0
lean & marbled	3½ oz.	18.0	290	0
Boston butt				
lean	3½ oz.	14.2	304	0
lean & marbled	3½ oz.	28.0	348	0
Canadian bacon, broiled	1 oz.	1.8	43	0
ham				
cured, butt, lean	3½ oz.	4.5	159	0
cured, butt, lean & marbled	3½ oz.	13.0	246	0
cured, canned	3 oz.	5.0	120	0
cured, shank, lean	3½ oz.	6.3	164	0
cured, shank, lean & marbled	2 slices	13.8	255	0
fresh, lean	3½ oz.	6.4	222	0
fresh, lean, marbled & fat	3½ oz.	18.3	306	0
ham loaf, glazed	3½ oz.	14.7	247	0
smoked	3½ oz.	7.0	140	0
smoked, 95% lean	3½ oz.	5.5	144	0
loin chop				
lean	1 chop	7.7	170	0
lean & fat	1 chop	22.5	314	0

Item	Serving	Total Fat (g)	Calories	Fiber (g)
picnic				
cured, lean	3½ oz.	9.9	211	0
fresh, lean	3½ oz.	7.4	150	0
shoulder, lean	2 slices	5.4	162	0
shoulder, marbled	2 slices	14.3	234	0
pig's feet, pickled	1 oz.	4.1	56	0
rib chop, trimmed	3½ oz.	9.9	209	0
rib roast, trimmed	3½ oz.	10.0	204	0
sausage				
brown and serve	1 oz.	9.4	105	0
patty	1	8.4	100	0
regular link	½ oz.	4.7	52	0
sirloin, lean, roasted	3½ oz.	10.2	207	0
spareribs roasted	6 medium	35.0	396	0
tenderloin, lean, roast	3½ oz.	4.8	155	0
top loin chop, trimmed	3½ oz.	7.7	193	0
top loin roast, trimmed	3½ oz.	7.5	187	0
processed meats				
bacon substitute				
(breakfast strips)	2 strips	4.8	50	0
beef, chipped	2 slices	1.1	47	0
beef breakfast strips	2 strips	7.0	100	0
beef jerky	1 oz.	3.6	90	0
bologna, beef/beef & pork	2 oz.	16.2	177	0
bratwurst				
pork	2 oz. link	22.0	256	0
pork & beef	2 oz. link	19.5	226	0
braunshweiger				
(pork liver sausage)	2 oz.	11.6	130	0
chicken roll	2 oz.	2.6	60	0
corn dog	1	20.0	330	0
corned beef, jellied	1 oz.	2.9	31	0
ham, chopped	1 oz.	2.3	55	0
hot dog/frank				
beef	1	13.2	145	0
chicken	1	8.8	116	0
97% fat-free varieties	1	1.6	55	0
turkey	1	8.1	102	0
kielbasa (Polish sausage)	1 oz.	8.3	80	0
knockwurst/knackwurst	2 oz. link	18.9	209	0
liver pâté, goose	1 oz.	12.4	131	0
pepperoni	1 oz.	13.0	140	0
salami				
cooked	1 oz.	10.0	116	0

Item	Serving	Total Fat (g)	Calories	Fiber (g)
dry/hard	1 oz.	10.0	120	0
sausage				
Italian	2 oz. link	17.2	216	0
90% fat-free varieties	2 oz.	4.6	86	0
Polish	2 oz. link	16.2	184	0
smoked	2 oz. link	20.0	229	0
Vienna	1 sausage	4.0	45	0
turkey breast, smoked	2 oz.	1.0	62	0
turkey ham	2 oz.	2.9	73	0
turkey loaf	2 oz.	1.0	62	0
turkey pastrami	2 oz.	3.5	80	0
turkey roll, light meat	2 oz.	4.1	83	0
turkey salami	2 oz.	7.8	110	0
veal				
arm steak				
lean	3½ oz.	4.8	180	0
lean & fat	3½ oz.	19.0	298	0
blade				
lean	3½ oz.	8.4	228	0
lean & fat	3½ oz.	16.6	276	0
breast, stewed	3½ oz.	18.6	256	0
chuck, med. fat, braised	3½ oz.	12.8	235	0
cutlet				
breaded	3½ oz.	15.0	319	0
round, lean	3½ oz.	12.8	194	0
round, lean & fat	3½ oz.	15.0	277	0
flank, med. fat, stewed	3½ oz.	32.0	390	0
foreshank, med. fat, stewed	3½ oz.	10.4	216	0
loin, med. fat, broiled	3½ oz.	13.4	234	0
loin chop				
lean	1 chop	4.8	149	0
lean & fat	3½ oz.	13.3	250	0
plate, med. fat, stewed	3½ oz.	21.2	303	0
rib chop				
lean	1 chop	4.6	125	0
lean & fat	1 chop	18.4	264	0
rump, marbled, roasted	3½ oz.	11.0	225	0
sirloin				
lean, roasted	3½ oz.	3.4	175	0
marbled, roasted	3½ oz.	6.5	181	0
sirloin steak				
lean	3½ oz.	6.0	204	0
lean & fat	3½ oz.	20.4	305	0

Item	Serving	Total Fat (g)	Calories	Fiber (g)
Milk and Yogurt				
buttermilk				
1% fat	1 cup	2.2	99	0
dry	1 T	0.4	25	0
choc. milk				
2% fat	1 cup	5.0	179	0
whole	1 cup	8.5	250	0
condensed milk, sweetened	½ cup	13.3	441	0
evaporated milk				
skim	½ cup	0.4	100	0
whole	½ cup	9.5	169	0
hot cocoa				
low cal, mix w/ water	1 cup	0.8	50	0
mix w/ water	1 cup	3.0	110	0
w/ skim milk	1 cup	2.0	158	0
w/ whole milk	1 cup	9.1	218	0
low-fat milk				
½% fat	1 cup	1.0	90	0
1% fat	1 cup	2.6	102	0
1.5% fat/acidophilus	1 cup	4.0	110	0
2% fat	1 cup	4.7	121	0
malted milk	1 cup	9.9	236	0
malt powder	1 T	1.6	86	0
milkshake				
choc. thick	1 cup	6.1	267	1
soft serve	1 cup	7.0	218	1
vanilla, thick	1 cup	6.9	255	0
skim milk				
liquid	1 cup	0.4	86	0
nonfat dry powder	¼ cup	0.2	109	0
whole milk				
3.5% fat	1 cup	8.2	150	0
dry powder	¼ cup	8.6	159	0
yogurt				
coffee/vanilla, low fat	1 cup	2.8	194	0
frzn, low fat	½ cup	3.0	115	0
frzn, nonfat	½ cup	0.2	81	0
fruit flavored, low fat	1 cup	2.6	225	0
plain				
low fat	1 cup	3.5	144	0

Item	Serving	Total Fat (g)	Calories	Fiber (g)
skim (nonfat)	1 cup	0.4	127	0
whole milk	1 cup	7.4	139	0

Miscellaneous

Item	Serving	Total Fat (g)	Calories	Fiber (g)
baking powder	1 t	0	3	0
baking soda	1 t	0	0	0
bouillon cube, beef or chicken	1	0.2	9	0
chewing gum	1 stick	0	10	0
choc., baking	1 oz.	15.7	148	1
cocoa, dry	⅓ cup	3.6	115	2
gelatin, dry	1 pkg.	0	23	0
honey	1 T	0	64	0
horseradish, prepared	1 t	0	2	0
icing, decorator	1 t	2.0	70	0
jam or jelly	1 T	0	50	0
marmalade, citrus	1 T	0	51	0
meat tenderizer	1 t	0	2	0
molasses	1 T	0	50	0
olives				
black	2 large	4.0	37	1
Greek	3 medium	7.1	67	1
green	2 medium	1.6	15	0
pickle relish				
chow chow	1 oz.	0.4	8	0
sweet	1 T	0.1	21	0
pickles				
bread & butter	4 slices	0.1	18	0
dill or sour	1 large	0.1	12	1
kosher	1 oz.	0.1	7	0
sweet	1 oz.	0.4	146	0
salt	1 t	0	0	0
spices/seasonings	1 t	0.2	5	0
sugar, all varieties	1 T	0	46	0
sugar substitutes	1 packet	0	4	0
syrup, all varieties	1 T	0	60	0

Item	Serving	Total Fat (g)	Calories	Fiber (g)
vinegar	1 T	0	2	0
yeast	1 T	0	23	0

Nuts and Seeds

Item	Serving	Total Fat (g)	Calories	Fiber (g)
almond paste	1 T	4.5	80	1
almonds	12–15	9.3	104	1
Brazil nuts	4 medium	11.5	114	1
cashews, roasted	6–8	7.8	94	2
chestnuts, fresh	3 small	0.8	66	4
coconut, dried, shredded	⅓ cup	9.2	135	1
hazelnuts (filberts)	10–12	10.6	106	1
macadamia nuts, roasted	6 medium	12.3	117	1
mixed nuts				
w/ peanuts	8–12	10.0	109	2
w/o peanuts	2 T	10.1	110	2
peanut butter, creamy or chunky	1 T	8.0	94	1
peanuts				
chopped	2 T	8.9	104	2
honey roasted	2 T	8.9	112	2
in shell	1 cup	17.7	209	3
pecans	2 T	9.1	90	1
pine nuts (pignoli)	2 T	9.1	85	2
pistachios	2 T	7.7	92	1
poppy seeds	1 T	3.8	44	1
pumpkin seeds	2 T	7.9	93	1
sesame nut mix	2 T	5.1	65	1
sesame seeds	2 T	8.8	94	1
sunflower seeds	2 T	8.9	102	1
trail mix w/ seeds, nuts, carob	2 T	5.1	87	1
walnuts	2 T	7.7	80	1

Pasta and Rice *(all measurements after cooking unless otherwise noted; 2 oz. uncooked pasta = ~ 1 cup cooked)*

Item	Serving	Total Fat (g)	Calories	Fiber (g)
macaroni				
semolina	1 cup	0.7	210	1
whole wheat	1 cup	2.0	210	5
noodles				
Alfredo	1 cup	29.7	462	3
cellophone, fried	1 cup	4.2	141	0
chow mein, canned	½ cup	8.0	150	0
egg	1 cup	2.4	212	1
manicotti	1 cup	1.0	210	1
ramen, all varieties	1 cup	8.0	190	1
rice	1 cup	0.3	140	1
romanoff	1 cup	23.0	372	3
rice				
brown	½ cup	0.6	116	2
fried	½ cup	7.2	181	1
long grain & wild	½ cup	2.1	120	2
pilaf	½ cup	7.0	170	1
Spanish style	½ cup	2.1	106	1
white	½ cup	1.2	111	0
spaghetti, enriched	1 cup	1.0	210	1

Poultry

Item	Serving	Total Fat (g)	Calories	Fiber (g)
chicken				
breast				
w/ skin, fried	½ breast	10.7	236	0
w/o skin, fried	½ breast	6.1	179	0
w/ skin, roasted	½ breast	7.6	193	0
w/o skin, roasted	½ breast	3.1	142	0
fryers				
w/ skin, batter dipped, fried	3½ oz.	17.4	289	0
w/o skin, fried	3½ oz.	11.1	237	0
w/ skin, roasted	3½ oz.	13.6	239	0
w/o skin, roasted	3½ oz.	7.4	190	0
giblets, fried	3½ oz.	13.5	277	0
gizzard, simmered	3½ oz.	3.7	153	0
heart, simmered	3½ oz.	7.9	185	0
leg				
w/ skin, fried	1 leg	8.7	120	0
w/ skin, roasted	1 leg	5.8	112	0
w/o skin, roasted	1 leg	2.5	76	0
liver, simmered	3½ oz.	5.5	157	0
roll, light meat	3½ oz.	7.4	159	0

Item	Serving	Total Fat (g)	Calories	Fiber (g)
stewers				
w/ skin	3½ oz.	18.9	285	0
w/o skin	3½ oz.	11.9	237	0
thigh				
w/ skin, fried	1 thigh	11.3	180	0
w/ skin, roasted	1 thigh	9.6	153	0
w/o skin, roasted	1 thigh	5.7	109	0
wing				
w/ skin, fried	1 wing	9.1	121	0
w/ skin, roasted	1 wing	6.6	99	0
duck				
w/ skin, roasted	3½ oz.	28.4	337	0
w/o skin, roasted	3½ oz.	11.2	201	0
pheasant, w/ or w/o skin, cooked	3½ oz.	9.3	181	0
quail, w/o skin, cooked	3½ oz.	9.3	213	0
turkey				
breast				
barbecued	3½ oz.	3.2	140	0
honey roasted	3½ oz.	2.8	112	0
oven roasted	3½ oz.	3.2	120	0
smoked	3½ oz.	3.5	112	0
dark meat				
w/ skin, roasted	3½ oz.	11.5	221	0
w/o skin, roasted	3½ oz.	7.2	187	0
ground	3½ oz.	13.3	219	0
ham, cured	3½ oz.	5.1	128	0
light meat				
w/ skin, roasted	3½ oz.	8.3	197	0
w/o skin, roasted	3½ oz.	3.2	157	0
loaf, breast meat	3½ oz.	1.6	110	0
patties, breaded/fried	1 patty	16.9	266	0
roll, light meat	3½ oz.	7.2	147	0
sausage, cooked	1 oz.	3.4	50	0

Salad Dressings

Item	Serving	Total Fat (g)	Calories	Fiber (g)
blue cheese				
fat free	1 T	0	10	0
low cal	1 T	1.9	27	0
regular	1 T	8.0	77	0
buttermilk, from mix	1 T	5.8	58	0
Caesar	1 T	7.0	70	0

Item	Serving	Total Fat (g)	Calories	Fiber (g)
French				
creamy	1 T	6.9	70	0
fat free	1 T	0	18	0
low cal	1 T	0.9	22	0
regular	1 T	6.4	67	0
garlic, from mix	1 T	9.2	85	0
Green Goddess				
low cal	1 T	2.0	27	0
regular	1 T	7.0	68	0
honey mustard	1 T	6.6	89	0
Italian				
creamy	1 T	5.5	54	0
fat free	1 T	0	6	0
low cal	1 T	1.5	16	0
regular zesty, from mix	1 T	9.2	85	0
Kraft, free	1 T	0	20	0
Kraft, reduced cal	1 T	1.0	25	0
mayonnaise type				
low cal	1 T	1.8	19	0
regular	1 T	4.9	57	0
oil & vinegar	1 T	7.5	69	0
ranch style, prep. w/ mayo	1 T	6.0	58	0
Russian				
low cal	1 T	0.7	24	0
regular	1 T	7.8	76	0
sesame seed	1 T	6.9	68	0
sweet & sour	1 T	0.9	29	0
Thousand Island				
fat free	1 T	0	20	0
low cal	1 T	1.6	24	0
regular	1 T	5.6	59	0
Snack Foods				
bagel chips or crisps	1 oz.	4.0	130	1
cheese straws	4 pieces	7.2	109	1
Cheetos Puffs	1 oz.	10.0	160	0
Chex snack mix, traditional	1 oz.	4	130	1

Item	Serving	Total Fat (g)	Calories	Fiber (g)
corn chips, Frito's				
barbecue	1 oz.	9.0	150	1
regular	1 oz.	10.0	160	1
corn nuts, all flavors	1 oz.	4.0	130	2
Cracker Jack	1 oz.	2.2	115	2
party mix (cereal, pretzels, nuts)	1 cup	23.0	312	3
popcorn				
air popped	1 cup	0.3	31	1
caramel	1 cup	4.5	150	1
microwave, "lite"	1 cup	1.0	27	1
microwave, plain	1 cup	3.0	47	1
microwave, w/ butter	1 cup	4.5	61	1
popped w/ oil	1 cup	3.1	55	1
pork rinds, Frito-Lay	1 oz.	9.3	151	0
potato chips				
individually	10 chips	8.0	113	0
baked, Lay's	1 oz.	1.5	110	2
by weight	1 oz.	11.2	159	1
barbecue flavor	1 oz.	9.5	149	1
potato sticks	1 oz.	10.2	152	0
pretzels	1 oz.	1.0	110	1
rice cakes	1	0	35	0
tortilla chips				
Doritos	1 oz.	6.6	139	1
no oil, baked	1 oz.	1.5	110	1
Tostitos	1 oz.	7.8	145	1

Soups

Item	Serving	Total Fat (g)	Calories	Fiber (g)
asparagus				
cream of, w/ milk	1 cup	8.2	161	1
cream of, w/ water	1 cup	4.1	87	1
bean				
w/ bacon	1 cup	5.9	173	4
w/ franks	1 cup	7.0	187	3
w/ ham	1 cup	8.5	231	3
w/o meat	1 cup	3.0	142	5
beef				
broth	1 cup	0.5	33	0
chunky	1 cup	5.1	171	2

Item	Serving	Total Fat (g)	Calories	Fiber (g)
beef barley	1 cup	1.1	72	1
beef noodle	1 cup	3.1	84	1
black bean	1 cup	1.5	116	2
broccoli, creamy w/ water	1 cup	2.8	69	1
Campbell's Healthy Request				
chicken, cream of, w/ water	1 cup	2.5	80	0
mushroom, cream of, w/ water	1 cup	3.0	70	0
tomato, w/ water	1 cup	2.0	90	0
canned vegetable type, w/o meat	1 cup	1.6	59	1
cheese w/ milk	1 cup	14.6	230	0
chicken				
chunky	1 cup	6.6	178	2
cream of, w/ milk	1 cup	11.5	191	0
cream of, w/ water	1 cup	7.4	116	0
chicken & dumplings	1 cup	5.5	97	0
chicken & stars	1 cup	1.8	55	1
chicken & wild rice	1 cup	2.3	76	1
chicken/beef noodle or veg.	1 cup	3.1	83	1
chicken gumbo	1 cup	1.4	56	1
chicken mushroom	1 cup	9.2	132	1
chicken noodle				
chunky	1 cup	5.2	149	2
w/ water	1 cup	2.5	75	0
chicken vegetable				
chunky	1 cup	4.8	167	2
w/ water	1 cup	2.8	74	1
chicken w/ noodles, chunky	1 cup	5.0	180	2
chicken w/ rice				
chunky	1 cup	3.2	127	2
w/ water	1 cup	1.9	60	1
clam chowder				
Manhattan chunky	1 cup	3.4	133	1
New England	1 cup	6.6	163	1
consommé w/ gelatin	1 cup	0	29	0
crab	1 cup	1.5	76	1

Item	Serving	Total Fat (g)	Calories	Fiber (g)
dehydrated				
bean w/ bacon	1 cup	3.5	105	2
beef broth cube	1 cube	0.3	6	0
beef noodle	1 cup	0.8	41	0
chicken, cream of	1 cup	5.3	107	1
chicken broth cube	1 cube	0.2	9	0
chicken noodle	1 cup	1.2	53	0
chicken rice	1 cup	1.4	60	0
clam chowder				
Manhattan	1 cup	1.6	65	1
New England	1 cup	3.7	95	0
minestrone	1 cup	1.7	79	0
mushroom	1 cup	4.9	96	0
onion				
dry mix	1 pkg.	2.3	115	1
prepared	1 cup	0.6	28	0
tomato	1 cup	2.4	102	0
vegetable beef	1 cup	1.1	53	0
gazpacho	1 cup	0.2	40	2
hmde or restaurant style				
beer cheese	1 cup	23.1	308	1
cauliflower, cream of				
w/ whole milk	1 cup	9.7	165	1
celery, cream of, w/ whole milk	1 cup	10.6	165	1
chicken broth	1 cup	1.4	38	0
clam chowder				
Manhattan	1 cup	2.2	76	2
New England	1 cup	14.0	271	1
corn chowder, traditional	1 cup	12.0	251	3
fish chowder, w/ whole milk	1 cup	13.5	285	1
gazpacho, traditional	1 cup	7.0	100	2
hot & sour	1 cup	7.1	134	1
mock turtle	1 cup	15.5	246	2
onion, French w/o cheese	1 cup	5.8	114	0
oyster stew, w/ whole milk	1 cup	17.7	268	0
seafood gumbo	1 cup	3.9	155	3
lentil	1 cup	1.0	161	3
minestrone				
chunky	1 cup	2.8	127	2
w/ water	1 cup	2.5	83	1
mushroom, cream of				
condensed	1 can	23.1	313	1

Item	Serving	Total Fat (g)	Calories	Fiber (g)
w/ milk	1 cup	13.6	203	1
w/ water	1 cup	9.0	129	1
mushroom barley	1 cup	2.3	76	1
mushroom w/ beef stock	1 cup	4.0	85	1
onion	1 cup	1.7	57	1
oyster stew, w/ water	1 cup	3.8	59	1
pea				
green, w/ water	1 cup	2.9	164	2
split	1 cup	0.6	58	1
split w/ ham	1 cup	4.4	189	1
potato, cream of				
w/milk	1 cup	7.4	157	2
shrimp, cream of, w/ milk	1 cup	9.3	165	1
tomato				
w/ milk	1 cup	6.0	160	1
w/ water	1 cup	1.9	86	0.5
tomato beef w/ noodle	1 cup	4.3	140	1
tomato bisque w/ milk	1 cup	6.6	198	1
tomato rice	1 cup	2.7	120	1
turkey, chunky	1 cup	4.4	136	2
turkey noodle	1 cup	2.0	69	1
turkey vegetable	1 cup	3.0	74	1
vegetable, chunky	1 cup	3.7	122	2
vegetable w/ beef, chunky	1 cup	3.0	134	2
vegetable w/ beef broth	1 cup	1.9	80	1
vegetarian vegetable	1 cup	1.2	73	1
wonton	1 cup	1.0	40	1

Vegetables

Item	Serving	Total Fat (g)	Calories	Fiber (g)
alfalfa sprouts, raw	½ cup	0.1	5	0
artichoke, boiled	1 medium	0.2	53	3
artichoke hearts, boiled	½ cup	0.1	37	3
asparagus, cooked	½ cup	0.3	22	2

Item	Serving	Total Fat (g)	Calories	Fiber (g)
avocado				
California	1 (6 oz.)	30.0	306	4
Florida	1 (11 oz.)	27.0	339	4
bamboo shoots, raw	½ cup	0.2	21	2
beans				
all types, cooked w/o fat	½ cup	0.4	143	9
baked, brown sugar & molasses	½ cup	1.5	132	4
baked, vegetarian	½ cup	0.6	118	5
baked w/ pork & tomato sauce	½ cup	1.3	123	5
homestyle, canned	½ cup	1.6	132	5
beets, pickled	½ cup	0.1	75	4
black-eyed peas(cowpeas), cooked	½ cup	0.6	100	2
broccoli				
cooked	½ cup	0.3	22	7
frzn, chopped, cooked	½ cup	0.1	25	2
frzn in butter sauce	½ cup	1.5	50	2
frzn w/ cheese sauce	½ cup	6.2	116	1
raw	½ cup	0.2	12	1
brussels sprouts, cooked	½ cup	0.4	30	2
butter beans, canned	½ cup	0.4	76	4
cabbage				
Chinese, raw	1 cup	0.2	10	2
green, cooked	½ cup	0.1	16	2
red, raw, shredded	½ cup	0.1	10	2
carrot				
cooked	½ cup	0.1	35	2
raw	1 large	0.1	31	2
cauliflower				
cooked	1 cup	0.2	30	3
frzn w/ cheese sauce	½ cup	4.8	75	1
raw	1 cup	0.1	12	4
celery				
cooked	½ cup	0.1	13	1
raw	1 stalk	0.1	6	1
chard, cooked	½ cup	0.1	18	2
chilies, green	¼ cup	0	10	0
Chinese-style vegetables, frzn	½ cup	4.0	74	3
chives, raw, chopped	1 T	0	1	0

Item	Serving	Total Fat (g)	Calories	Fiber (g)
collard greens, cooked	½ cup	0.1	13	2
corn				
corn on the cob	1 medium	1.0	120	4
cream style, canned	½ cup	0.5	93	4
frzn, cooked	½ cup	0.1	67	4
frzn w/ butter sauce	½ cup	2.2	110	3
whole kernel, cooked	½ cup	1.1	89	5
cucumber				
w/ skin	½ medium	0.2	20	1
w/o skin, sliced	½ cup	0.1	7	0
dandelion greens, cooked	½ cup	0.3	17	2
eggplant, cooked	½ cup	0.1	13	2
endive lettuce	1 cup	0.2	8	1
garbanzo beans (chick peas), cooked	½ cup	2.1	135	5
green beans				
french style, cooked	½ cup	0.2	26	2
snap, cooked	½ cup	0.2	22	2
hominy, white or yellow, cooked	1 cup	0.7	138	3
Italian-style vegetables, frzn	½ cup	5.5	102	2
kale, cooked	½ cup	0.3	21	2
kidney beans, red, cooked	½ cup	0.5	112	8
leeks, chopped, raw	¼ cup	0.1	16	1
lentils, cooked	½ cup	0.4	116	8
lettuce, leaf	1 cup	0.2	10	1
lima beans, cooked	½ cup	0.4	108	5
miso (soybean product)	½ cup	8.4	284	4
mushrooms				
canned	½ cup	0.2	19	1
fried/sautéed	4 medium	7.4	90	1
raw	½ cup	0.2	9	1
mustard greens, cooked	½ cup	0.2	11	2
okra, cooked	½ cup	0.1	25	3
onions				
canned, french fried	1 oz.	15.0	175	0
chopped, raw	½ cup	0.1	30	1

Item	Serving	Total Fat (g)	Calories	Fiber (g)
parsley, chopped, raw	¼ cup	0.1	5	0
parsnips, cooked	½ cup	0.2	63	3
peas, green, cooked	½ cup	0.2	67	4
pepper, bell, chopped, raw	½ cup	0.1	13	2
pimentos, canned	1 oz.	0	10	0
potato				
au gratin				
from mix	½ cup	6.0	140	2
hmde	½ cup	9.3	160	1
baked w/ skin	1 medium	0.2	220	4
boiled w/o skin	½ cup	0.1	116	2
french fries				
frzn	10 pieces	4.4	111	2
hmde	10 pieces	8.3	158	1
hash browns	½ cup	10.9	163	2
knishes	1	3.2	73	1
mashed				
from flakes, w/ milk & marg.	½ cup	6.0	130	1
w/ milk & marg.	½ cup	4.4	111	1
pan fried, O'Brien	½ cup	15.0	231	3
potato pancakes	1 cake	12.6	237	1
potato puffs, frzn, prep. w/ oil	½ cup	11.6	183	3
scalloped				
from mix	1 serving	5.9	127	1
hmde	½ cup	4.8	105	1
w/ cheese	½ cup	9.7	177	1
twice-baked potato, w/ cheese	1 medium	11.8	370	4
pumpkin, canned	½ cup	0.3	41	4
radish, raw	10	0.2	7	1
rhubarb, raw	1 cup	0.2	29	2
sauerkraut, canned	½ cup	0.2	22	4
scallions, raw	5 medium	0.2	60	4
soybeans, mature, cooked	½ cup	7.7	149	4
spinach				
cooked	½ cup	0.2	21	3
creamed	½ cup	5.1	79	3
raw	1 cup	0.2	12	3
squash				
acorn				
baked	½ cup	0.1	57	4

Item	Serving	Total Fat (g)	Calories	Fiber (g)
mashed w/o fat	½ cup	0.1	41	3
butternut, cooked	½ cup	0.1	41	4
summer				
cooked	½ cup	0.3	18	2
raw, slice	½ cup	0.1	13	1
winter, cooked	½ cup	0.6	39	4
succotash, cooked	½ cup	0.8	111	3
sweet potato				
baked	1 small	0.1	118	7
candied	½ cup	3.4	144	5
mashed w/o fat	½ cup	0.5	172	5
tempeh (soybean product)	½ cup	6.4	165	1
tofu (soybean curd), raw	4 oz.	5.4	90	1
tomato				
boiled	½ cup	0.5	32	1
raw	1 medium	0.4	26	1
stewed	½ cup	0.2	34	1
tomato paste, canned	½ cup	1.2	110	4
turnip greens, cooked	½ cup	0.2	15	2
turnips, cooked	½ cup	0.1	14	2
water chestnuts, canned, sliced	½ cup	0	35	1
watercress, raw	½ cup	0	2	0
wax beans, canned	½ cup	0.2	25	2
yam, boiled/baked	½ cup	0.1	79	3
zucchini, cooked	½ cup	0.1	14	2

Vegetable Salads

Item	Serving	Total Fat (g)	Calories	Fiber (g)
Caesar salad w/o anchovies	1 cup	7.2	80	1
carrot-raisin salad	½ cup	5.8	153	4
chef salad w/o dressing	1 cup	4.2	65	1
coleslaw				
w/ mayo-type dressing	½ cup	14.2	147	1
w/ vinaigrette	½ cup	3.0	78	1
gelatin salad w/ fruit & cheese	½ cup	4.6	74	0
macaroni salad w/ mayo	½ cup	12.8	200	1
pasta primavera salad	1 cup	5.9	149	3

Item	Serving	Total Fat (g)	Calories	Fiber (g)
potato salad				
German style	½ cup	3.5	140	1
w/ mayo dressing	½ cup	11.5	189	1
salad bar items				
alfalfa sprouts	2 T	0	2	0
bacon bits	1 T	1.0	21	0
beets, pickled	2 T	0	18	0
broccoli, raw	2 T	0	3	0
carrots, raw	2 T	0	6	0
cheese, shredded	2 T	4.6	56	0
chickpeas	2 T	0.3	36	1
cottage cheese	½ cup	5.1	116	0
croutons	½ oz.	2.6	62	0
cucumber	2 T	0	2	0
eggs, cooked, chopped	2 T	1.9	27	0
lettuce	½ cup	0	4	0
mushrooms, raw	2 T	0	2	0
onion, raw	2 T	0.1	7	0
pepper, green, raw	2 T	0	3	0
potato salad	½ cup	10.3	179	0
tomato, raw	2 slices	0	2	0
seven-layer salad	1 cup	17.8	226	2
tabbouli salad	½ cup	9.5	173	3
taco salad w/ taco sauce	1 cup	14.0	202	2
three-bean salad	½ cup	8.2	145	3
three-bean salad, w/o oil	½ cup	0.2	90	3
Waldorf salad w/mayo	½ cup	12.7	157	2

Appendix B

BODY MASS INDEX

The body mass index (BMI) provides information about the health risks of your weight. It is calculated as weight in kilograms divided by height in squared meters.*

Adult Weight Classifications	BMI
Underweight	<18.5
Normal (Healthy)	18.5–24.9
Overweight	25.0–29.9
Obese	≥30

The following formula can be used to calculate the BMI using pounds and inches:

$$\text{BMI} = \frac{\text{(Weight in pounds)}}{\text{(Height in inches)(Height in inches)}} \times 703$$

A person who weighs 188 pounds and is 5 feet 10 inches tall has a BMI of 27:

$$\frac{\text{(188 lbs.)}}{\text{(70 inches)(70 inches)}} \times 703 = 27$$

* Source: Centers for Disease Control and Prevention (CDC), Alanta, GA.

As the BMI goes above the normal range, the risk of diseases such as type 2 diabetes, heart disease, and certain cancers increases. To find what is considered a normal (healthy) weight range for any height, find your height (in inches) in the left column of the Body Mass Index Table on the following page, and slide your finger along the row, under the numbers 19 to 25 (Normal) in the BMI row at the top of the table.

BODY MASS INDEX TABLE

	Normal						Overweight					Obese										
BMI	19	20	21	22	23	24	25	26	27	28	29	30	31	32	33	34	35	36	37	38	39	40
Height (inches)								**Body Weight (pounds)**														
58	91	96	100	105	110	115	119	124	129	134	138	143	148	153	158	162	167	172	177	181	186	191
59	94	99	104	109	114	119	124	128	133	138	143	148	153	158	163	168	173	178	183	188	193	196
60	97	102	107	112	118	123	128	133	138	143	148	153	158	163	168	174	179	184	189	194	199	204
61	100	106	111	116	122	127	132	137	143	148	153	158	164	169	174	180	185	190	195	201	206	211
62	104	109	115	120	126	131	136	142	147	153	158	164	169	175	180	186	191	196	202	207	213	218
63	107	113	118	124	130	135	141	146	152	158	163	169	175	180	186	191	197	203	208	214	220	225
64	110	116	122	128	134	140	145	151	157	163	169	174	180	186	192	197	204	209	215	221	227	232
65	114	120	126	132	138	144	150	156	162	168	174	180	186	192	198	204	210	216	222	228	234	240
66	118	124	130	136	142	148	155	161	167	173	179	186	192	198	204	210	216	223	229	235	241	247
67	121	127	134	140	146	153	159	166	172	178	185	191	198	204	211	217	223	230	236	242	249	255
68	125	131	138	144	151	158	164	171	177	184	190	197	203	210	216	223	230	236	243	249	256	262
69	128	135	142	149	155	162	169	176	182	189	196	203	209	216	223	230	236	243	250	257	263	270
70	132	139	146	153	160	167	174	181	188	195	202	209	216	222	229	236	243	250	257	264	271	278
71	136	143	150	157	165	172	179	186	193	200	208	215	222	229	236	243	250	257	265	272	279	286
72	140	147	154	162	169	177	184	191	199	206	213	221	228	235	242	250	258	265	272	279	287	294
73	144	151	159	166	174	182	189	197	204	212	219	227	235	242	250	257	265	272	280	288	295	302
74	148	155	163	171	179	186	194	202	210	218	225	233	241	249	256	264	272	280	287	295	303	311
75	152	160	168	176	184	192	200	208	216	224	232	240	248	256	264	272	279	287	295	303	311	319
76	156	164	172	180	189	197	205	213	221	230	238	246	254	263	271	279	287	295	304	312	320	328

Source: Adapted from *Clinical Guidelines on the Identification, Evaluation, and Treatment of Overweight and Obesity in Adults: The Evidence Report*, CDC

Resources

REFERENCES

Bailey, D. G., and Dresser, G. K. 2004. Interactions between grapefruit juice and cardiovascular drugs. *American Journal of Cardiovascular Drugs* 4(5):281–97.

Church, T. S., Thomas, D. M., Tudor-Locke, C., Katzmarzyk, P. T., Earnest, C. P., et al. 2011. Trends over 5 decades in U.S. occupation-related physical activity and their associations with obesity. *PloS One* 6(5):e19657. doi:10:1371

Dallman, M. F. 2010. Stress-induced obesity and the emotional nervous system. *Trends in Endocrinology and Metabolism* 21(3):159–65.

Hill, James O., and Wing, R. 2003 (Summer). Weight management and obesity symposium. *Permanente Journal* 7(3):34–37.

Pope, Jamie, and Katahn, Martin. 2006. *The T-Factor Fat Gram Counter.* New York: W. W. Norton.

Rolls, Barbara J., and Barnett, Robert A. 2000. *The Volumetrics Weight Control Plan.* New York: HarperCollins.

Weeks, Kent M. 2004. *A Leaner America.* Bloomington, IN: Xlibris.

We Rate the Hot Diets. 2011 (June). Pick your ideal diet. *Consumer Reports* 76(6):14–16.

BIBLIOGRAPHY

Anderson, Bob, and Anderson, Jean. 2010. *Stretching: 30th Anniversary Edition.* Bolinas, CA: Shelter Publications.

Austin, Denise. 2004. *Sculpt Your Body with Balls and Bands.* New York: Rodale Books.

Hill, James O., and Peters, John C., with Jortberg, Bonnie T. 2004. *The Step Diet.* New York: Workman Publishing.

Katch, Frank I., and Katch, Victor L., with Brown, Gene. 2000. *The Fidget Factor: The Easy Way to Burn Up to 1000 Extra Calories Every Day.* Kansas City: Stonesong Press.

Kessler, David A. 2009. *The End of Overeating.* New York: Rodale.

Laughlin, Terry, with Delves, John. 1996. *Total Immersion.* New York: Simon and Schuster.

Netzer, Corinne T. 2009. *The Complete Book of Food Counts.* New York: Dell.

Sobel, David, and Klein, Arthur C. 1995. *Arthritis: What Exercises Work.* New York: St. Martin's Griffin.

Wilkins, F., and Wilkins, D. 2011. *DietMinder: Personal Food and Fitness Journal.* Eugene, OR: MemoryMinder Journals.

INSTRUCTIONAL DVDS AND CDS

Anh-Huong, Nguyen, and Hanh, Thich Nhat. 2006. *Walking Meditation.* Boulder, CO: Sounds True.

Bodhipaksa. 2002. *Guided Meditations.* Newmarket, NH: Wildmind Meditation.

Kessler, David A. 2009. *The End of Overeating.* New York: Simon and Schuster.

Lam, Paul. 1995. *Tai Chi: 6 Forms, 6 Easy Lessons.* New York: East Acton Videos.

Lam, Paul. 1998. *Tai Chi for Older Adults.* New York: East Acton Videos.

Lam, Paul. 1999. *Tai Chi: The 24 Forms.* New York: East Acton Videos.

WEIGHT MANAGEMENT AT VANDERBILT UNIVERSITY

Weight-management classes at Vanderbilt University are offered at the Kim Dayani Health Promotion Center, 1500 Medical Center Drive, Nashville, TN 37232. Telephone 615-322-4751. www.vanderbilthealth.com/dayani.

WEBSITES

There is a wealth of information about diet, nutrition, and physical activity on the web. Here are some suggestions to get you started if you want to do more research. Website addresses are current as of this writing.

The following websites offer practical information on diet, nutrition, and/or activity. Some focus on a particular health concern to which obesity contributes.

American Academy of Pediatrics: www.aap.org

American Association for Cancer Research: www.aacr.org

American Diabetes Association: www.diabetes.org

American Dietetic Association: www.eatright.org

American Heart Association: www.americanheart.org

American Medical Association: www.ama-assn.org

American Obesity Association: www.obesity.org

Center for Science in the Public Interest: www.cspinet.org

Centers for Disease Control and Prevention: www.cdc.gov

Health Finder: www.healthfinder.gov

Healthy People 2010: www.healthypeople.gov

InteliHealth: www.intelihealth.com

Mayo Clinic: www.mayoclinic.com

MedlinePlus health information: www.nlm.nih.gov/medlineplus

National Cancer Institute: www.nci.nih.gov

National Heart, Lung, and Blood Institute: www.nhlbi.nih.gov
National Institute of Child Health and Human Development:
www.nichd.nih.gov
National Institute of Diabetes and Digestive and Kidney Diseases:
www.niddk.nih.gov
National Weight Control Registry: www.nwcr.ws
President's Council on Fitness, Sports, and Nutrition: www.fitness.gov
United States Department of Agriculture (USDA): www.usda.gov

The following websites are good places to purchase fitness equipment and accessories.

Academy Sports + Outdoors: www.academy.com
Active Living Now: www.activelivingnow.com
Amazon.com: www.amazon.com
Walgreens (online store): www.walgreens.com

The following websites are geared for tracking diet, activity levels, or giving weight-management advice. Some require you to join their online community. Some cost a small fee.

America On the Move: www.americaonthemove.org
Calorie Counter: www.caloriesperhour.com
Cyberdiet: www.cyberdiet.com
FitDay: www.fitday.com
FitnessOnline: www.fitnessonline.com
Fitness Partner: www.primusweb.com/fitnesspartner
GymAmerica: www.gymamerica.com
Web Fitness Tools: www.webfitnesstools.com

These websites are directed to children, with interactive games to facilitate learning about health.

Dole 5-a-Day: www.dole.com/#/superkids
KidsHealth: www.kidshealth.org

These websites offer information about nutrition in our schools.

American School Food Service Association: www.asfsa.org

Parent Teacher Association (PTA): www.pta.org

USDA Healthy School Meals Resource System:
www.schoolmeals.nal.usda.com

USDA Team Nutrition: www.fns.usda.gov

These websites offer information about eating disorders.

Academy for Eating Disorders: www.aedweb.org

Weight.com: www.weight.com

For more information on the benefits of physical activity, take a look at these websites.

National Association for Sport and Physical Education: www.aahperd.org

National Center for Chronic Disease Prevention and Health Promotion:
www.cdc.gov/nccdphp

Shape Up America!: www.shapeup.org

Here are a few websites that offer good pedometers to help in tracking your activity level.

Accusplit: www.accusplit.com

New Lifestyles: www.new-lifestyles.com

Walk4Life: www.walk4life.com

To find calorie counts of some meals served at many chain restaurants across the country, try the following websites. Be aware, however, that their idea of a low-calorie or low-fat-gram count might be a lot higher than you would want for weight loss or even maintenance.

www.healthydiningfinder.com

www.dietriot.com/fff

www.fatcalories.com

THE ROTATION DIET POCKET EDITION FOR WOMEN

You can average a weight loss of up to a pound a day for twenty-one days if you follow the menus as they are laid out on pages 369–75. Best results are obtained with few substitutions. If a particular food does not agree with you, please read Chapter 7 concerning allowable substitutions.

Recipes and other suggestions for food preparation are found in Chapter 7. I have not given the names of specific recipes here, as I did in the Chapter 7 menus, but there are recipes in Chapter 7 for the foods marked with an asterisk.

To be sure that everyone can follow the Rotation Diet and never feel hungry, I have designed an insurance policy that will enable you to overcome temptations and still achieve close-to-optimum results. It has two clauses. The first is called *free vegetables*. Should any temptations to deviate from the diet arise during the twenty-one days of the diet, you can eat unlimited quantities of free vegetables with any meal and at any time of the day as snacks (see page 375 of this Pocket Edition). Free vegetables contain almost no calories. In addition, you can choose *safe fruits* (see page 376 of this Pocket Edition). Safe fruits, while they contain a few more calories than free vegetables, are additional insurance against ever being hungry. They can also be used as a source of quick energy whenever you need it, and will hardly slow your weight loss.

You can photocopy the Pocket Edition of the Rotation Diet so that you can carry it with you for ready reference. In case a photocopier is not available, you can cut out the Pocket Edition pages without damaging the other contents of the book.

COUPLES CAN USE THE
ROTATION DIET TOGETHER

See the text of the Pocket Edition menus for women (Weeks 1 and 2), or see page 87 of Chapter 7.

If you show the Rotation Diet to your friends and they wish to use it, please have them read Chapters 1, 7, and 8 before they start. (Be sure to read these chapters yourself before you start.)

THE COMPLETE ROTATION DIET
PLAN MENUS FOR WOMEN

The Rotation Diet is designed to be used with the special recipes that are available for items marked with an asterisk (see Chapter 7 menus for specific names of recipes, or leaf through recipes). However, you can prepare everything in your own way provided you do not use any fat in preparation except where indicated.

Also, you can use the portion sizes below as a guide when eating out during this period. *Weights below are all cooked weights.* See Chapter 7 for information on shrinkage to be expected during cooking. No-cal salad dressings can be used at any time, so they are not always indicated. Note: tablespoon and teaspoon measures are level measures.

WEEK 1

In the case of couples who wish to use the Rotation Diet together, men may use the basic Week 1 diet plan for women with the addition of all of the following each day:

2 more grain servings (bread, cereal, or crackers)
50 percent larger portions of meat, fish, or fowl
1 tablespoon of butter, oil, or regular salad dressing
3 safe fruits

The calorie goal for men is 1200 calories for the first three days, and 1500 calories for the next four. Additional information on serving sizes, *with calorie values,* can be found with the recipes in Chapter 7.

Day 1

Breakfast	½ grapefruit, 1 slice of whole-wheat bread,* 1 ounce of cheese, no-cal beverage
Lunch	2 ounces of salmon* (canned in water), unlimited free vegetables, 5 whole-wheat crackers, no-cal beverage
Dinner	3 ounces of baked chicken,* 1 cup of cauliflower,* ½ cup of beets,* 1 apple, no-cal beverage

Day 2

Breakfast   ½ banana, 1 ounce of high-fiber cereal, 8 ounces of skim or low-fat milk, no-cal beverage

Lunch   4 ounces of low-fat cottage cheese,* unlimited free vegetables, 1 slice of whole-wheat bread,* no-cal beverage

Dinner   3 ounces of poached fish fillet,* 1 cup of broccoli,* ½ cup of carrots,* ½ grapefruit, no-cal beverage

Day 3

Breakfast   1 slice of whole-wheat bread,* 1 tablespoon of peanut butter, 1 apple, no-cal beverage

Lunch   2 ounces of water-packed tuna* or 3 medium sardines,* 5 whole-wheat crackers, unlimited free vegetables, no-cal beverage

Dinner   3 ounces of beefsteak* or hamburger patty,* 1 cup of asparagus,* 1 cup of dinner salad,* 1 ounce of cheese, 1 orange, no-cal beverage

Day 4

Breakfast   ½ banana, 1 ounce of high-fiber cereal, 8 ounces of skim or low-fat milk, no-cal beverage

Lunch   2 ounces of water-packed tuna,* unlimited free vegetables, 2 slices of whole-wheat bread,* 1 teaspoon of mayonnaise or lo-cal dressing,* ½ grapefruit, no-cal beverage

Dinner   3 ounces of baked chicken,* ½ cup of carrots,* 1 cup of dinner salad,* 1 ounce of cheese, 1 apple, no-cal beverage

Day 5

Breakfast   1 cup of berries, 4 ounces of low-fat cottage cheese,*
            5 whole-wheat crackers, no-cal beverage

Lunch   3 medium sardines* or 2 ounces of water-packed
            tuna,* unlimited free vegetables, 2 slices of whole-
            wheat bread,* 1 teaspoon of mayonnaise or lo-cal
            dressing,* ½ grapefruit, no-cal beverage

Dinner   3 ounces of beefsteak* or hamburger patty,* ½ cup of
            green beans,* 1 cup of broccoli,* 1 ounce of cheese, 1
            apple, no-cal beverage

Day 6

Breakfast   ½ cantaloupe, 1 ounce of cheese, 1 slice of whole-
            wheat bread,* no-cal beverage

Lunch   1 hard-boiled egg,* unlimited free vegetables, 2 slices
            of whole-wheat bread,* 1 teaspoon of mayonnaise or
            low-cal salad dressing,* ½ grapefruit, no-cal beverage

Dinner   3 ounces of fish fillet,* 1 cup of asparagus,* ½ cup of
            green peas,* 1 apple, no-cal beverage

Day 7

Breakfast   ½ banana, 1 ounce of high-fiber cereal, 8 ounces of
            skim or low-fat milk, no-cal beverage

Lunch   1 cup of berries, 4 ounces of low-fat cottage cheese,*
            2 slices of whole-wheat bread,* no-cal beverage

Dinner   3 ounces of baked chicken,* 1 cup of cauliflower,* ½
            cup of carrots,* 1 apple, no-cal beverage

WEEK 2

In Week 2 you may add a mid-morning, a mid-afternoon, and an evening snack, intentionally incorporating three servings of your *safe fruit*. It is not obligatory to include all of these snacks in addition to the menus below, but they are permitted within the 1200-calorie limits for this week. You may also add 1 tablespoon of butter, margarine, oil, or regular salad dressing to your diet each day. Use it for cooking or as a spread.

For couples' use, men should add all of the following each day to the daily menus of the Rotation Diet for women, below.

2 more grain servings (bread, cereal, or crackers)
50 percent larger portions of vegetables and main courses

Optional for men: another tablespoon of fat for spread or seasoning. The calorie goal for males is 1800 per day throughout Week 2. Additional information on serving sizes, *with calorie values*, can be found with the recipes in Chapter 7.

Day 8

Breakfast   ½ grapefruit, 1 slice of whole-wheat bread,* 1 tablespoon of peanut butter, 8 ounces of skim or low-fat milk, no-cal beverage

Lunch   large (2 cups) fruit salad,* 1 ounce of cheese, 5 whole-wheat crackers, no-cal beverage

Dinner   4½ ounces of salmon steak*, ½ cup of peas and baby onions,* 1 cup of dinner salad,* no-cal beverage

Day 9

Breakfast   ½ banana, 1 ounce of high-fiber cereal, 8 ounces of skim or low-fat milk, no-cal beverage

Lunch   large chef salad* (1 ounce of turkey and 1 ounce of cheese, plus salad vegetables), 5 whole-wheat crackers, lo-cal dressing,* no-cal beverage

Dinner   4½ ounces of baked chicken,* 1 small (3½-ounce) baked potato, 1 cup of green beans,* 1 ounce of cheese, 1 apple, no-cal beverage

Day 10

Breakfast   1 cup of sliced fruit, 4 ounces of low-fat cottage cheese,* 1 slice of whole-wheat bread,* no-cal beverage

Lunch   sandwich* (2 ounces of meat or cheese), unlimited free vegetables, 1 orange, no-cal beverage

Dinner   2 cups of stir-fry vegetables,* ½ cup of brown or wild rice,* 2 tablespoons of grated cheese, 1 apple, no-cal beverage

Day 11

Breakfast   1 cup of fresh pineapple (or other fresh fruit), 1 ounce of cheese, 1 slice of whole-wheat bread,* no-cal beverage

Lunch   large (2–3 cups), spinach salad,* lo-cal dressing,* 1 apple or pear, 1 ounce of cheese, no-cal beverage

Dinner   6 ounces of steak,* 1 small (3½-ounce) baked potato, 1 cup of braised carrots and celery,* ½ grapefruit, no-cal beverage

Day 12

Breakfast   ½ cup of sliced fruit for cereal, 1 ounce of high-fiber cereal, 8 ounces of skim or low-fat milk, no-cal beverage

Lunch   3 ounces of water-packed tuna or 4–5 medium sardines,* unlimited free vegetables plus sliced tomato and green peppers, lo-cal dressing,* 1 slice of whole-wheat bread,* no-cal beverage

Dinner   6 ounces of lean pork chop* (or other lean meat), ½ baked acorn squash,* 1 cup of broccoli,* ½ grapefruit, no-cal beverage

Day 13

Breakfast   ½ melon, 1 hard- or soft-boiled egg, 1 slice of whole-wheat bread,* no-cal beverage

Lunch   4½-ounce ground-beef patty,* 4 ounces of low-fat cottage cheese,* sliced tomato and unlimited free vegetables, lo-cal dressing,* no-cal beverage

Dinner   1 cup of pasta (choice of sauces),* 2 tablespoons of Parmesan cheese, 1 cup of dinner salad,* choice of 1 fresh fruit for dessert, no-cal beverage

Day 14

Breakfast   ½ grapefruit, 1 cup of oatmeal, 2 tablespoons of raisins, dash of cinnamon, 4 ounces of skim or low-fat milk, no-cal beverage

Lunch   toasted open-faced sandwich* or regular sandwich* (2 ounces of meat or cheese), unlimited free vegetables, 1 cup of assorted sliced fresh fruit, no-cal beverage

Dinner   4 ounces of pot roast* (including vegetables), 1 cup of dinner salad,* lo-cal dressing,* 1 ounce of cheese, 1 apple, no-cal beverage

WEEK 3

Repeat the menus of Week 1, or use the Alternate Menus in Chapter 11 for the 600- and 900-calorie rotations.

When you finish your twenty-one days on the Rotation Diet, BE VERY SURE THAT YOU FOLLOW MY DIRECTIONS FOR MAKING A TRANSITION TO MAINTENANCE IN WEEK 4 (CHAPTER 9).

UNLIMITED FREE-VEGETABLE LIST

You can eat all you want of the vegetables on this list at any time. They provide many vitamins and minerals, together with beneficial amounts of fiber, with virtually no calories. Eat them plain or use only no-cal salad dressings (your choice, or see page 119 of the Rotation Diet).

asparagus	chard	radishes
bamboo shoots	collard greens	spinach
broccoli	cucumber	summer squash
brussels sprouts	lettuce	tomatoes
cabbage	green beans	turnip greens
carrots	kale	water chestnuts
cauliflower	mushrooms	wax beans
celery	onions	zucchini

SAFE-FRUIT LIST

Choose safe fruits from this list when you need a lift, feel intolerably hungry, or are tempted to deviate from your diet for any reason, and you don't think the free vegetables will fill the bill. Carry one with you at all times as a snack.

apples	oranges
berries	peaches
grapefruit	pears
grapes	pineapple
melons	tangerines

Whenever you are tempted to deviate from the Rotation Diet, make a safe-fruit substitution instead. This ensures that you will achieve close to the maximum possible weight loss.

THE ROTATION DIET POCKET EDITION FOR MEN

You can average a weight loss of up to a pound a day for twenty-one days if you follow the menus as they are laid out on pages 379–85. Best results are obtained with few substitutions. If a particular food does not agree with you, please read Chapter 7 concerning allowable substitutions.

Recipes and other suggestions for food preparation are found in Chapter 7. I have not given the names of specific recipes here, as I did in the Chapter 7 menus, but there are recipes in Chapter 7 for the foods marked with an asterisk.

To be sure that everyone can follow the Rotation Diet and never feel hungry, I have designed an insurance policy that will enable you to overcome temptations and still achieve close-to-optimum results. It has two clauses. The first is called *free vegetables*. Should any temptations to deviate from the diet arise during the twenty-one days of the diet, you can eat unlimited quantities of free vegetables with any meal and at any time of the day as snacks (see page 385 of this Pocket Edition). Free vegetables contain almost no calories. In addition, you can choose *safe fruits* (see page 386 of this Pocket Edition). Safe fruits, while they contain a few more calories than free vegetables, are additional insurance against ever being hungry. They can also be used as a source of quick energy whenever you need it, and will hardly slow your weight loss.

You can photocopy the Pocket Edition of the Rotation Diet so that you can carry it with you for ready reference. In case a photocopier is not available, you can cut out the Pocket Edition pages without damaging the other contents of the book.

COUPLES CAN USE THE ROTATION DIET TOGETHER

See the text at the beginning of the Pocket Edition menus for women (Weeks 1 and 2), or see page 87 of Chapter 7.

If you show the Rotation Diet to your friends and they wish to use it, please have them read Chapters 1, 7, and 8 before they start. (Be sure to read these chapters yourself before you start.)

THE COMPLETE ROTATION DIET PLAN MENUS FOR MEN

The Rotation Diet is designed to be used with the special recipes that are available for items marked with an asterisk (see Chapter 7 menus for specific names of recipes, or leaf through recipes). However, you can prepare everything in your own way provided you do not use any fat in preparation except where indicated, or as part of the amount permitted in the next paragraph. Also, you can use the portion sizes below as a guide when eating out during this period. *Weights below are all cooked weights.* See Chapter 7 for information on shrinkage to be expected during cooking.

Men may add 1 tablespoon of butter, margarine, or regular salad dressing to each day's menu and remain within the calorie limits. No-cal salad dressings can be used at any time, so they are not always indicated. Note: tablespoon and teaspoon measures are level measures.

WEEK 1

Day 1

Breakfast ½ banana, 1 ounce of high-fiber cereal, 8 ounces of skim or low-fat milk, no-cal beverage

Lunch large chef salad* (1 ounce each of cheese and turkey, plus any salad vegetables), lo-cal dressing,* 5 whole-wheat crackers, no-cal beverage

Dinner 4½ ounces of baked chicken,* 1 small (3½-ounce) baked potato, 1 cup of green beans,* 1 apple, 1 ounce of cheese, no-cal beverage

Day 2

Breakfast ½ grapefruit, 1 slice of whole-wheat bread,* 1 tablespoon of peanut butter, 8 ounces of skim or low-fat milk, no-cal beverage

Lunch large (2 cups) fruit salad,* 1 ounce of cheese, 5 whole-wheat crackers, no-cal beverage

Dinner 6 ounces of fish fillets,* ½ cup of peas and baby onions,* 1 cup of dinner salad,* lo-cal dressing,* no-cal beverage

Day 3

Breakfast	1 cup of sliced fruit (your choice), 4 ounces of low-fat cottage cheese,* 1 slice of whole-wheat bread,* no-cal beverage
Lunch	combination sandwich* (2 ounces of meat or cheese), unlimited free vegetables, 1 orange, no-cal beverage
Dinner	*2 cups of stir-fry vegetables,** ½ cup of brown or wild rice,* 2 tablespoons of grated cheese, 1 apple, no-cal beverage

Day 4

Breakfast	1 cup of berries, 1½ ounces of high-fiber cereal, 8 ounces of skim or low-fat milk, 1 slice of whole-wheat bread,* 1 teaspoon of preserves, no-cal beverage
Lunch	large (2–3 cups) spinach salad,* lo-cal dressing,* 5 whole-wheat crackers, 1 apple or pear, no-cal beverage
Dinner	½ grapefruit, 6 ounces of steak,* 1 small (3½-ounce) baked potato, 1 cup of braised carrots and celery,* no-cal beverage

Day 5

Breakfast	½ melon, 1 hard- or soft-boiled egg, 2 slices of whole-wheat bread,* 1 teaspoon of preserves, no-cal beverage
Lunch	4½-ounce ground-beef patty,* 4 ounces of low-fat cottage cheese,* unlimited free vegetables, 1 slice of whole-wheat bread,* 1 serving of fruit (your choice), no-cal beverage

Dinner   1 cup of pasta (choice of sauces),* 4 tablespoons of Parmesan cheese, 1 cup of dinner salad,* lo-cal dressing,* ½ grapefruit, no-cal beverage

Day 6

Breakfast   1 cup of sliced fruit, 1½ ounces of high-fiber cereal, 1 slice of whole-wheat bread,* 8 ounces of skim or low-fat milk, no-cal beverage

Lunch   4–5 medium sardines or 3 ounces of water-packed tuna,* unlimited free vegetables plus sliced tomato and green pepper, lo-cal dressing,* 2 slices of whole-wheat bread,* no-cal beverage

Dinner   6 ounces of lean pork chop* (or other lean meat), ½ baked acorn squash,* 1 cup of broccoli,* 1 slice of whole-wheat bread,* ½ grapefruit, no-cal beverage

Day 7

Breakfast   ½ grapefruit, 1 cup of oatmeal, 2 tablespoons of raisins, dash of cinnamon, 4 ounces of skim or low-fat milk, no-cal beverage

Lunch   open-faced sandwich* (2 portions with 1 ounce of cheese and sliced tomato, or see lunch sandwich Day 3), unlimited free vegetables, lo-cal dressing,* 1 cup of assorted fresh fruit, no-cal beverage

Dinner   4 ounces of pot roast* (including vegetables), 1 cup of dinner salad,* lo-cal dressing,* 1 apple, no-cal beverage

WEEK 2

Day 8

Breakfast   ½ melon, 2 slices of whole-wheat bread,* 2 ounces of cheese, no-cal beverage

Lunch   tuna-salad sandwich* (3 ounces of water-packed tuna), unlimited free vegetables, 1 serving of fruit (your choice), no-cal beverage

Dinner   6 ounces of baked chicken,* ½ cup of spinach and broccoli casserole* (or 1 cup of broccoli*), ½ baked acorn squash,* 1 apple, 1 ounce of cheese (if casserole recipe is not used), no-cal beverage

Day 9

Breakfast   1 cup of oatmeal, 2 tablespoons of raisins, dash of cinnamon, 4 ounces of skim or low-fat milk, 1 slice of whole-wheat bread,* 1 teaspoon of preserves, no-cal beverage

Lunch   large (2 cups) fruit salad,* 4 ounces of low-fat cottage cheese,* 5 whole-wheat crackers, no-cal beverage

Dinner   6 ounces of fish fillet,* ½ baked tomato,* 1 small (3½-ounce) baked potato, 1 cup of dinner salad,* 1 ounce of cheese, 1 apple, no-cal beverage

Day 10

Breakfast   1 orange, 2 slices of whole-wheat bread,* 2 ounces of cheese, no-cal beverage

Lunch   tuna salad* (3 ounces of water-packed tuna) on greens with sliced tomatoes and green pepper, plus unlimited free vegetables, lo-cal dressing,* no-cal beverage

Dinner 6 ounces of steak,* 1 cup of stir-fry spinach,* 1 small (3½-ounce) baked potato with cottage cheese dressing* (or 2 tablespoons of sour cream), choice of 1 fruit, no-cal beverage

Day 11

Breakfast ½ melon, 4 ounces of low-fat cottage cheese,* 1 slice of whole-wheat bread,* 1 teaspoon of preserves, no-cal beverage

Lunch sandwich* (2 ounces of meat or cheese), unlimited free vegetables, lo-cal dressing,* no-cal beverage

Dinner 6 ounces of baked salmon,* ½ cup of peas and baby onions,* 1 cup of dinner salad,* lo-cal dressing,* choice of 1 fruit, 1 ounce of cheese, no-cal beverage

Day 12

Breakfast ½ grapefruit, 2 slices of whole-wheat bread,* 1 tablespoon of peanut butter, 1 teaspoon of preserves, no-cal beverage

Lunch 1 cup of soup (commercial or see Soups*), 10 whole-wheat crackers, 2 ounces of cheese, unlimited free vegetables, lo-cal dressing,* no-cal beverage

Dinner eggplant casserole* (1 serving, or 6-ounce serving of lean meat of your choice*), ½ cup of carrots,* 1 cup of dinner salad,* lo-cal dressing,* 1 apple, no-cal beverage

Day 13

Breakfast   1 cup of berries, 1½ ounces of high-fiber cereal, 1 slice of whole-wheat bread,* 1 teaspoon of preserves, 8 ounces of skim or low-fat milk, no-cal beverage

Lunch   large chef salad* (1 ounce each of turkey and cheese, plus salad vegetables), lo-cal dressing,* 5 whole-wheat crackers, no-cal beverage

Dinner   6 ounces of baked chicken,* ½ cup of brown or wild rice,* 1 cup of broccoli,* 1 ounce of cheese, 1 apple, no-cal beverage

Day 14

Breakfast   1 cup of sliced fruit, 4 ounces of low-fat cottage cheese,* 1 slice of whole-wheat bread,* 1 teaspoon of preserves, no-cal beverage

Lunch   sandwich* (2 ounces of meat or cheese), unlimited free vegetables, lo-cal dressing,* ½ grapefruit, no-cal beverage

Dinner   6 ounces of baked or broiled fish,* ½ baked tomato,* 1 cup of green beans with chives,* 1 slice of whole-wheat bread,* 1 ounce of cheese, 1 fruit of your choice, no-cal beverage

WEEK 3

Repeat the menus of Week 1, or use the Alternate Menus in Chapter 11 for the 1200- and 1500-calorie rotations.

When you finish your twenty-one days on the Rotation Diet, BE VERY SURE THAT YOU FOLLOW MY DIRECTIONS FOR MAKING A TRANSITION TO MAINTENANCE IN WEEK 4 (CHAPTER 9).

UNLIMITED FREE-VEGETABLE LIST

You can eat all you want of the vegetables on this list at any time. They provide many vitamins and minerals, together with beneficial amounts of fiber, with virtually no calories. Eat them plain or use only no-cal salad dressings (your choice, or see page 119 of the Rotation Diet).

asparagus	chard	radishes
bamboo shoots	collard greens	spinach
broccoli	cucumber	summer squash
brussels sprouts	lettuce	tomatoes
cabbage	green beans	turnip greens
carrots	kale	water chestnuts
cauliflower	mushrooms	wax beans
celery	onions	zucchini

SAFE-FRUIT LIST

Choose safe fruits from this list when you need a lift, feel intolerably hungry, or are tempted to deviate from your diet for any reason, and you don't think the free vegetables will fill the bill. Carry one with you at all times as a snack.

apples	oranges
berries	peaches
grapefruit	pears
grapes	pineapple
melons	tangerines

Whenever you are tempted to deviate from the Rotation Diet, make a safe-fruit substitution instead. This ensures that you will achieve close to the maximum possible weight loss.

INDEX

Page numbers in **boldface** refer to recipes.

acorn squash, **137**
activity, physical, 14
    author's personal experience with,
        174–76, 179–81, 207
    best time for, 165–66
    calories burned in, 163, 165, 167,
        169–72, 179–81, 183
    cardiovascular endurance increased
        by, 172–73
    choosing form of, 173–74
    exercise equipment for, 181–82, 186
    length of sessions, 177
    in long-term weight management,
        161–87
    in maintenance period, 198
    metabolic rate and, 19–21, 22,
        24–25, 26–27, 177–79
    overall goal for, 162–65
    in Rotation Diet, 45
    as stress reduction, 231
    see also walking
adolescents, Rotation Diet
    inappropriate for, 17
aerobic dance, 168, 185
Agriculture Department, U.S.
    (USDA), 22, 84
alcohol consumption, 306n
almond chicken, **126**
America on the Move (website), 297

Anderson, Bob, 187
Anderson, Jean, 187
Andrew (40-year-old man), 218–19
appetite, 188–89
    stimulated by "supernormal" foods,
        49–52, 55–57, 223–25
apple-nut bran squares, **292**
arthritis, 16, 44, 187
Arthritis: What Exercises Work (Sobel
    and Klein), 186–87
artichoke-stuffed portobellos, **265**
asparagus:
    caraway, **138**
    cold Dijon, **138**
Austin, Denise, 182

baked:
    chicken, **127–28**
    fish fillets, **132**
    fish in spring herbs, **267**
    lemon-, chicken, **128**
    rainbow trout, **132–33**
    tomato, **146**
ballroom dancing, 168
balsamic no-cal dressing, **120**
barley, vegetable soup with, **261–62**
bean spread, Mexican, **111**
beef:
    marinated flank steak, **122–23**

beef (*continued*)
  pepper burgers, **277**
  pot roast of, **125–26**
  steak and hamburger teriyaki style,
    120–21
  steak flamed in brandy, **121**
beets, gingered, **139–40**
beverages:
  allowable in Rotation Diet, 76–77
  calorie, fat gram, and fiber counter
    for, 306
bicycling, 168
bingeing, 189
blood sugar levels, 16
Bodhipaksa, 231
body mass index, 357–58
  table for, 359
Bonnie (success story), 208–9
Bragg Liquid Aminos soy sauce, 282
bran, apple-nut squares, **292**
bread pudding, **293**
breads, 102, **103–5**
  calorie, fat gram, and fiber counter
    for, 307–10
  oatmeal batter, **104–5**
  whole-wheat batter, **103–4**
breakfast cakes, whole-wheat, **296**
Breakstone's Lowfat Cottage Cheese,
    108
broccoli, 140, **140–41**
  with black olives, **140–41**
  cauliflower soup, **259**
  and spinach casserole, **144–45**
broiled:
  rainbow trout, **132–33**
  snapper, **267–68**
burgers, pepper beef, **277**
Bush, Milt, 175–76
B vitamins, 154

Caesar salad, spinach, **264**
cake, poppy-seed, **294**
calcium, 154
calorie, fat gram, and fiber counter,
    303–56
calories, 23*n*
  in body fat, 190
  burned at rest, 24
  burned in physical activity, 163, 165,
    167, 169–72, 179–81, 183
  in free vegetables, 73–74
  increased intake of, in maintenance
    period, 191–92, 194
  needed to maintain weight, 22–23,
    26
  in safe fruits, 73, 74–75
  in sandwiches, 109
candy, 52–53
  calorie, fat gram, and fiber counter
    for, 310–12
  see also chocolate
cardiovascular disease, 16
cardiovascular endurance, 172–73
carrots, **141–42**
  and celery, braised, **142**
  citrus, **287**
  a l'orange, **141**
  with onions, **141**
case histories, *see* success stories
casseroles:
  medley, **273–74**
  spinach, stovetop, **290**
  spinach and broccoli, **144–45**
  vegetarian eggplant, **134**
cauliflower:
  broccoli soup, **259**
  savory steamed, **142**
celery and carrots, braised, **142**
Center for Human Nutrition, 164

cereals, 106
    calorie, fat gram, and fiber counter
        for, 312–14
cheese(s), 107
    calorie, fat gram, and fiber counter
        for, 314–15
    toast, Mexican, **107–8**
    see also cottage cheese
chef salad, creative, **115**
chicken, **126–29**
    almond, **126**
    baked, **127–28**
    lemon-baked, **128**
    Mrs. Dash crunchy popcorn, **275**
    and mushrooms, Mrs. Dash
        country, **274**
    paprika, **268**
    sesame, **268–69**
    slim Southern-style fried, **284**
    and Swiss salad, **262–63**
    teriyaki, **269**
    Tomasi, **129**
chickpea-tuna salad, **285–86**
children, Rotation Diet inappropriate
        for, 17
Chinese fried rice, **286**
chocolate, 52, 53
cholesterol, 15–16
citrus carrots, **287**
clam:
    and garlic sauce, **135–36**
    mushroom chowder, **260–61**
coffee, 77
combination foods: calorie, fat gram,
        and fiber counter for, 315–20
Complete Book of Food Counts, The
        (Netzer), 305
Consumer Reports, 56
cottage cheese:

plus, **108**
    salad dressing, **118**
couples, Rotation Diet for, 83–84
crabmeat spread, **110**
crackers, 102, 105
    toasted oat thins, **295–96**
curried:
    lentils, **270–71**
    unstuffed hard-boiled egg, **108–9**

Davis, Dr. (author's pediatrician),
        29–30
Delves, John, 184
depression, 16
desserts, **292–94**
    apple-nut bran squares, **292**
    bread pudding, **293**
    pineapple ice, **293–94**
    poppy-seed cake, **294**
    and toppings: calorie, fat gram, and
        fiber counter for, 320–24
diabetics, 16, 56
Dietary Guidelines for Americans
        (2010), 54, 55, 153
diet dinners, frozen, 36
diet drinks, 151–52
*DietMinder: Personal Food and Fitness
        Journal* (MemoryMinder
        Journals), 221
Dijon asparagus, cold, **138**
dill, salmon with, **280**
dinner salad, **115–16**
diuretic foods, 197–98
diuretics, 16
dried fruits, 152
Dunkin' Donuts, 54–55

eating diaries, 220–21
eating out, 61

eating out (*continued*)
  strategies for, 36–37, 65–67, 228
  by women on Rotation Diet, 66
egg(s):
  calorie, fat gram, and fiber counter
    for, 325
  curried unstuffed hard-boiled,
    108–9
  drop soup, **260**
eggplant casserole, vegetarian, **134**
1800-calorie rotation menus, 253–58
electrolyte balance, 17, 80
elliptical trainers, 168
End of Overeating, The (Kessler), 218
energy balance, 23–24
Estimates of Energy Requirements
  (EER), 22–23
exercise equipment, 181–82, 186

family cooperation:
  in Rotation Diet, 61, 62–65, 85–86
  working mothers and, 68
fantasy, in mastery of eating situations,
  225, 226–29
fast foods, 304–5
  calorie, fat gram, and fiber counter
    for, 325–27
fat, body, 19, 201
  calories in, 190
  excess storage of, 163, 200
fat, dietary, 200
  calorie, fat gram, and fiber counter
    for, 327–28
  metabolic rate and, 19, 26,
    200–201
fat gram, calorie, and fiber counter,
  303–56
fever, 51
fiber, 201–2

fiber, calorie, and fat gram counter,
  303–56
*Fidget Factor, The: The Easy Way to Burn
  Up to 1000 Extra Calories Every
  Day* (Frank I. and Victor L.
  Katch), 180–81
fidgeting, 180–81
1500-calorie rotation menus, 249–52
fish, **130–33**
  baked in spring herbs, **267**
  baked or broiled rainbow trout,
    132–33
  broiled snapper, **267–68**
  calorie, fat gram, and fiber counter
    for, 328–32
  crabmeat spread, **110**
  fillets, **132**
  fillets, poached, **130–31**
  halibut steak with vegetables, **271**
  luncheon tuna vinaigrette, **118**
  royal Indian salmon, **133**
  salmon loaf, **279**
  salmon with dill, **280**
  salmon with herbs, **116**
  sardines vinaigrette, **117**
  seafood Italia, **280–81**
  sesame scallops, **281**
  shrimp and snow peas, **282**
  shrimp jambalaya, **283**
  standard portions of, 78–79
  tuna-chickpea salad, **285–86**
  tuna or salmon salad, **116**
  tuna- or salmon-salad sandwich,
    111
flexibility exercises, 186–87
Food and Drug Administration, 84
fowl:
  calorie, fat gram, and fiber counter
    for, 345–46

standard portions of, 78–79
see also chicken
free vegetables, 45, 59, 153
    as allowable deviations from
        Rotation Diet, 56, 69, 70
    calories in, 73–74
    list of, 73–74
fruit(s):
    calorie, fat gram, and fiber counter
        for, 332–34
    dried, 152
    puff, German, **295**
    salad, creative, **114**
    see also safe fruits
fruit juice:
    calorie, fat gram, and fiber counter
        for, 334–35
    undiluted, 152

garlic and clam sauce, **135–36**
German fruit puff, **295**
gingered beets, **139–40**
Goo Goo Clusters, 53
goulash, paprika pork, **276**
grains:
    standard portions of, 79
    see also rice
grapefruit:
    possible drug interaction of, 76
    as safe fruit, 69–70, 75
gravies, sauces, and dips: calorie, fat
        gram, and fiber counter for,
        335–37
green beans:
    almondine, **138–39**
    with chives, **139**
    spicy, **289–90**
Guided Meditations CD (Bodhipaksa),
    231

halibut steak with vegetables, **271**
hamburger and steak teriyaki style,
    120–21
Health and Human Services,
    Department of (HHS), 22
Healthy Choice entrées, 36
herb(s):
    baked fish in spring, **267**
    salmon with, **116**
herbed pork, 123–24
herb salt, 81, **147–48**
Hill, James O., 164, 228
hypertension, 16–17, 30, 38, 56,
    82–83, 231

ice, pineapple, **293**
imagination, in mastery of eating
        situations, 225, 226–29
iron, 154

"Jenny Craig at Home" (*Consumer
        Reports*), 56
junk food, 13–14, 56
    on family menus, 64–65
    nutrients vs. calories in, 229–30
    "supernormal" status of, 14, 55–56

Kaplan, Gordon, 39–40
Katch, Frank I., 180, 181
Katch, Victor L., 180, 181
Katherine (success story), 210–12,
    217–18, 219
Kessler, David A., 218, 219
Kim Dayani Health Promotion
    Center, 41
Klein, Arthur C., 187

Lam, Paul, 231
lamb chops, **124**

Laughlin, Terry, 184
Lean Cuisine entrées, 36
lemon-baked chicken, **128**
lentils, curried, **270–71**
Lisa (success story), 212–15
lo-cal salad dressing, **119**
low-fat milk, 106

main courses, **265–86**
   artichoke-stuffed portobellos, **265**
   Asian stir-fry, **266**
   baked fish in spring herbs, **267**
   broiled snapper, **267–68**
   chicken paprika, **268**
   chicken sesame, **268–69**
   chicken teriyaki, **269**
   curried lentils, **270–71**
   halibut steak with vegetables, **271**
   lean and perfect pizza, **272–73**
   medley casserole, **273–74**
   Mrs. Dash country chicken and
      mushrooms, **274**
   Mrs. Dash crunchy popcorn
      chicken, **275**
   paprika pork goulash, **276**
   pepper beef burgers, **277**
   quick skillet (pork), **278**
   salmon loaf, **279**
   salmon with dill, **280**
   seafood Italia, 280–81
   sesame scallops, **281**
   shrimp and snow peas, **282**
   shrimp jambalaya, **283**
   slim Southern-style fried chicken,
      284
   spicy orange pork, **284–85**
   tuna-chicken salad, **285–86**
maintenance period, 188–202
   alternate menus for, 232–33

   calorie intake in, 191–92, 194
   guidelines for, summarized, 192,
      199
   increasing food intake in, 193–95
   increasing metabolic needs in,
      200–201
   naturally diuretic foods in, 197–98
   physical activity in, 198
   safe fruits in, 199
   salt intake in, 195–96
   snacks in, 189, 190
   water consumption in, 198
   water retention and, 189–92
marinated flank steak, **122–23**
meat:
   calorie, fat gram, and fiber counter
      for, 337–41
   sauce, **136**
   spread, **110**
   standard portions of, 78–79
   see also beef; pork
medley casserole, **273–74**
men:
   alternate maintenance menus for,
      233, 234, 235–58
   calories needed by, 22–23
   complete Rotation Diet plan menus
      for, 94–101
   family cooperation and, 63
   portion size for, 79
   shopping lists for, 160
metabolic rate:
   dietary fat and, 19, 26, 200–201
   effect of weight loss on, 27
   effects of food on, 25–26
   energy balance and, 23–24
   of fat vs. muscle tissue, 26
   physical activity and, 19–21, 22,
      24–25, 26–27, 177–79

Rotation Diet and, 28
  starvation response and, 27–28
  200-calorie solution and, 19–28
Mexican bean spread, **111**
Mexican cheese toast, **107–8**
milk and milk products, 106–8
  calorie, fat gram, and fiber counter
    for, 342–43
  standard portions of, 79
minerals, 17, 154–55
mineral supplements, 153–55
minitrampolines, 168
miscellaneous food items: calorie, fat
    gram, and fiber counter for,
    343–44
Morning-Star Farms Grillers Original,
    36
Mrs. Dash:
  country chicken and mushrooms,
    274
  crunchy popcorn chicken, **275**
  low-salt seasoning, 82
muscles, 178–79
mushroom(s):
  artichoke-stuffed portobellos, **265**
  clam chowder, **260–61**
  Mrs. Dash country chicken and, **274**

National Institute of Mental Health,
    40
National Weight Control Registry
    (NWCR), 15, 54, 64, 228
  website, 297
  weight loss strategies, summary of,
    204–6
Netzer, Corrine T., 305
Nguyen Anh-Huong, 231
nibbling while preparing meals, 223
900-calorie rotation menus, 238–41

no-cal salad dressing, **119**
  balsamic, **120**
no-salt seasoning, **148**
nursing mothers, Rotation Diet
    inappropriate for, 17
nuts and seeds: calorie, fat gram, and
    fiber counter for, 344

oatmeal batter bread, **104–5**
oat thins, toasted, **295–96**
olives, black, broccoli with, **140–41**
onions:
  baby, peas and, **143–44**
  carrots with, **141**
orange pork, spicy, **284–85**
oven-fried potatoes, **287**

paprika:
  chicken, **268**
  pork goulash, **276**
pasta:
  calorie, fat gram, and fiber counter
    for, 344–45
  garlic and clam sauce for,
    135–36
  meat sauce for, **136**
Pavlov, Ivan, 51
peas:
  and baby onions, **143–44**
  old thymey, **143**
  shrimp and snow peas, **282**
pepper beef burgers, **277**
Pilates, 174
pineapple ice, **293**
pizza, lean and perfect, **272–73**
poached fish fillets, **130–31**
Pocket Edition of Rotation Diet:
  for men, 377–86
  for women, 367–76

polenta:
  basic, **288**
  seasoned, **289**
poppy-seed cake, **294**
pork:
  goulash, paprika, **276**
  herbed, **123–24**
  quick skillet, **278**
  spicy orange, **284–85**
potassium, 17
potato(es):
  oven-fried, **287**
  salad, **263**
pot roast of beef, **125–26**
pregnant women, Rotation Diet
    inappropriate for, 17
pulse rate, 171–73

racquetball, 168
racquet sports, 168
rainbow trout, baked or broiled,
    132–33
recipes, **101–48, 259–96**
Recommended Dietary Allowances
    (RDAs), 17, 80, 84, 153, 155,
    229, 230
rehearsal of eating situations,
    226–29
RESPeRATE (breathing relaxation
    device), 231
restaurants and dieting, *see* eating out
resting energy expenditure (REE), 24,
    26, 28
Rhonda (success story), 215–17
rice:
  brown or wild, **144**
  calorie, fat gram, and fiber counter
    for, 344–45
  Chinese fried, **286**

Rotation Diet:
  alternate menus for, 232–58
  author's personal success with,
    29–37
  average weight loss in, 9–10, 73
  beverages allowed in, 76–77
  combining meals in, 149–50
  for couples, 83–84
  deviations from, 58
  dieters' reactions to, 46–47
  family cooperation in, 61, 62–65,
    85–86
  first clinical trial of, 46
  food preparation in, 77–78, 234–35
  food variety beneficial in, 148–49
  general instructions for, 12–15,
    72–73
  getting started on, 61–71
  menus for men in, 94–101
  menus for women in, 87–94
  metabolic rate and, 28
  nutritional value of, 153
  physical activity in, 45
  physician consulted before start of,
    16–17
  Pocket Edition of, for men, 377–86
  Pocket Edition of, for women,
    367–76
  recipes for, **101–48, 259–96**
  research in development of, 39–46
  reversing order of meals in, 149–50
  "safe foods" and, 69–71
  salt use in, 81
  serving sizes in, 77–79
  shopping lists for, 155–60
  for singles, 84–85
  skipping meals in, 149–50
  special health benefits of, 15–18
  substitutions in, 80, 148–49

temptations removed from home in,
    62–65
vacation from, *see* maintenance
    period
vegetarian substitutions in, 150–51
rowing, 168
RYVITA Dark Rye crackers, 105
RYVITA Sesame Rye crackers, 105

safe fruits, 45, 153
    as allowable deviation from
        Rotation Diet, 56, 59, 69–71
    calories in, 73, 74–75
    choosing of, 74–76
    list of, 76
    in maintenance period, 199
    as snacks, 75–76, 79–80, 230
salad dressings, **118–20**
    balsamic no-cal, **120**
    calorie, fat gram, and fiber counter
        for, 346–47
    cottage-cheese, **118**
    lo-cal, **119**
    no-cal, **119**
salads, **114–18**
    chicken and Swiss, **262–63**
    chickpea-tuna, **285–86**
    creative chef, **115**
    creative fruit, **114**
    dinner, **115–16**
    luncheon tuna vinaigrette, **118**
    potato, **263**
    salmon with herbs, **116**
    sardines vinaigrette, **117**
    seasoned tomato, **263**
    spinach, **117**
    spinach Caesar, **264**
    tuna-chickpea, **285–86**
    tuna or salmon, **116**

salmon:
    with dill, **280**
    with herbs, **116**
    loaf, **279**
    royal Indian, **133**
    salad, **116**
    salad sandwich, **111**
salt, 81–83
    foods high in, 81
    herb, 81, **147–48**
    hypertension and, 16, 38, 82–83
    water retention caused by, 11, 81,
        191
sandwiches, 109
    calories in, 109
    combination, **109**
    crabmeat spread for, **110**
    meat spread for, **110**
    Mexican bean spread for, **111**
    tuna or salmon-salad, **111**
sardines vinaigrette, **117**
sauces:
    calorie, fat gram, and fiber counter
        for, 335–37
    garlic and clam, **135–36**
    meat, **136**
scallops, sesame, **281**
Sculpt Your Body with Balls and Bands
    (Austin), 182
seafood:
    Italia, **280–81**
    see also fish
serving sizes, 77–79
sesame:
    chicken, **268–69**
    scallops, **281**
shopping lists:
    for men's menus, 160
    for women's menus, 155–59

shrimp:
  jambalaya, **283**
  and snow peas, **282**
singles, Rotation Diet for, 84–85
600-calorie rotation menus, 235–37
600/900 calorie rotation:
  nutritional value of, 153
  snacks in, 79–80
  vegetable preparation in, 137
sleep apnea, 16
Smart Ones entrées, 36
snacks:
  calorie, fat gram, and fiber counter
    for, 347–48
  free vegetables as, 79–80
  in maintenance period, 189, 190
  safe fruits as, 75–76, 79–80, 230
snapper, broiled, **267–68**
snow peas and shrimp, **282**
Sobel, Dava, 187
sodium, 17, 82–83, 191–92
  foods high in, 81, 195–96
soups, **112–14, 259–62**
  base for, **112–13**
  broccoli-cauliflower, **259**
  calorie, fat gram, and fiber counter
    for, 348–51
  egg drop, **260**
  mushroom clam chowder, **260–61**
  vegetable, Thursday's, **113–14**
  vegetable, with barley, **261–62**
South Beach Living entrées, 36
Southern-style fried chicken, **284**
soy sauce, 81, 191
spicy green beans, **289–90**
spicy orange pork, **284–85**
spinach:
  and broccoli casserole, **144–45**
  Caesar salad, **264**

casserole, stovetop, **290**
salad, **117**
stir-fry, **145**
spreads:
  crabmeat, **110**
  meat, **110**
  Mexican bean, **111**
starvation response, 27–28
steak:
  flamed in brandy, **121**
  flank, marinated, **122–23**
  and hamburger teriyaki style,
    120–21
stir-fry:
  Asian, **266**
  spinach (or other greens), **145**
  vegetables, **146–47**
stovetop spinach casserole, **230**
strength training, 186
stress reduction, 230–31
Stretching: 30th Anniversary Edition
    (Anderson and Anderson), 187
stretching exercises, 187
success stories, 208–17
  Bonnie, 208–9
  Katherine, 210–12, 217–18, 219
  Lisa, 212–15
  Rhonda, 215–17
  Tracy, 210
succotash, **291**
sugar, 151–53
supernormal foods, 14, 49–52, 55–57,
    58, 203, 220
  controlling your response to,
    223–26
  stress reduction and, 230
sweeteners, artificial, 151, 152
swimming, 167–68, 183–85
Swiss and chicken salad, **262–63**

Tai Chi, 174, 185, 231
Tai Chi for Older Adults DVD (Lam), 231
Tai Chi: 6 Forms 6 Easy Lessons DVD (Lam), 231
Tai Chi: The 24 Forms DVD (Lam), 231
Tarpley, Ed, 32, 175
tea, 77
  herb, 77
Tennessean, 40, 53
tennis, 168
  as author's physical activity, 175–76
teriyaki:
  chicken, **269**
  steak and hamburger, **120–21**
Thera-Band Progressive Resistance Exercise Bands, 182
thermic effect of food (TEF), 25–26
Thich Nhat Hanh, 231
thrombophlebitis, 31, 32
tomato:
  baked, **146**
  salad, seasoned, **263**
Total Immersion (Laughlin and Delves), 184
Tracy (success story), 210
triglycerides, 15–16
Triscuit Hint of Salt, 105
Tums tablets, 154
tuna:
  -chickpea salad, **285–86**
  luncheon, vinaigrette, **118**
  salad, **116**
  salad sandwich, **111**
1200-calorie rotation menus, 242–48

Unsalted Tops Saltines, 105

Vanderbilt Weight Management Program (WMP), 11–13, 21, 23, 28, 32, 40, 57, 149, 151, 173, 205, 220
  original program of, 41–43
  Rotation Diet developed in, 39–46
  weight loss in, 9
varicose veins, 31
vegetables, **137–47**
  acorn squash, **137**
  baked tomato, **146**
  braised carrots and celery, **142**
  broccoli with black olives, **140–41**
  brown or wild rice, **144**
  calorie, fat gram, and fiber counter for, 351–55
  calories in, 137
  caraway asparagus, **138**
  carrots a l'orange, **141**
  carrots with onions, **141**
  Chinese fried rice, **286**
  citrus carrots, **287**
  cold Dijon asparagus, **138**
  gingered beets, **139–40**
  green beans almondine, **138–39**
  green beans with chives, **139**
  halibut steak with, **271**
  old thymey peas, **143**
  oven-fried potatoes, **287**
  peas and baby onions, **143–44**
  polenta, basic, **288**
  polenta, seasoned, **289**
  savory steamed cauliflowerets, **142**
  soup, Thursday's, **113–14**
  soup with barley, **261–62**
  spicy green beans, **289–90**
  spinach and broccoli casserole, **144–45**
  spinach salad, **117**

vegetables (*continued*)
  standard portions of, 78
  stir-fry, **146–47**
  stir-fry spinach (or other greens),
    145
  stovetop spinach casserole, **290**
  succotash, **291**
vegetable salads: calorie, fat gram, and
    fiber counter for, 355–56
vegetarian:
  eggplant casserole, **134**
  substitutions, 150–51
vitamins, 17, 154–55
vitamin supplements, 153–55

walking, 173
  calories burned in, 10–11, 165, 167,
    169, 171–72
  maintaining motivation for,
    166–67
  setting goals for, 163–65
  for weight control, 20–21
Walking Meditation CD (Nguyen Anh-
    Huong and Thich Nhat Hanh),
    231
walking shoes, 183
Wallston, Ken, 40
water, drinking of, 76, 198
water aerobics, 184–85
water retention:
  during maintenance period, 189–92
  salt or sodium intake and, 11, 81,
    191
  by women, 9
weight loss:
  effect on metabolism of, 27
  NWCR strategies for, 204–6
  weight maintenance and, 10–11

weight management, 47–48
  body mass index (BMI) and, 357–59
  building confidence in, 57–60
  dietary challenges and, 217–19
  eating-diaries useful in, 220–21
  eating habits and, 221–22
  fantasy or imagination in, 225,
    226–29
  fundamentals of, 220–21
  identifying problem areas in,
    222–26
  junk food and, 55–56, 229–30
  Lisa's 20 rules for, 213–15
  long-term weight maintenance,
    203–31
  maintaining exercise program in,
    67–68
  motivation and, 206–7
  original Vanderbilt program of,
    41–43
  rehearsal in, 226–29
  stress reduction in, 230–31
  success stories, 208–17
  see also "supernormal" foods
Weingartner, Joyce, 102
whole wheat:
  batter bread, **103–4**
  breakfast cakes, **296**
WMP, *see* Vanderbilt Weight
    Management Program
women:
  alternate maintenance menus for,
    233, 235–58
  calories needed by, 22–23
  complete Rotation Diet plan menus
    for, 87–94
  in early WMP programs, 44–46
  eating out by, 66

family cooperation needed by,
    63–65, 68
portion size for, 78–79
shopping lists for, 155–59

World Health Organization, 50

yoga, 174
yogurt, 106